Sex on Your Terms

Sex on Your Terms

What to Say
— to explain your limits
— to repel sexual pressure
— to avoid being falsely accused
— to escape disease

Elizabeth Powell
St. Louis Community College at Meramec

Allyn and Bacon
Boston • London • Toronto • Sydney • Tokyo • Singapore

Vice President, Publisher: Social Sciences: Susan Badger
Executive Editor: Laura Pearson/Sean Wakely
Marketing Manager: Joyce Nilsen
Senior Production Administrator: Marjorie Payne
Editorial Assistant: Jennifer Normandin
Cover Administrator: Suzanne Harbison
Composition/Prepress Buyer: Linda Cox
Manufacturing Buyer: Aloka Rathnam
Editorial-Production Service: Chestnut Hill Enterprises, Inc.

Copyright © 1996 by Allyn & Bacon
A Simon & Schuster Company
Needham Heights, Massachusetts 02194

Library of Congress Cataloging-in-Publication Data

Powell, Elizabeth
    Sex on your terms : what to say--to explain your limits, to repel sexual pressure, to avoid being falsely accused, to escape disease / by Elizabeth Powell.
      p. cm.
    Includes bibliographical references and index.
    ISBN 0-205-17925-8 (alk. paper)
    1. Communication in sex. 2. Assertiveness (Psychology) 3. Sexual harassment--Prevention. 4. Acquaintance rape--Prevention.
5. Sexually transmitted diseases--Prevention. I. Title.
HQ23.P66 1995
613.9′6--dc20
                                          95-23581
                                          CIP

Printed in the United States of America

10 9 8 7 6 5 4 3 2 1   00 99 98 97 96 95

In memory of my great-grandmother, Eliza Davis,
who survived rape in the aftermath of the Civil War,
this offering for Justice

For all survivors of sexual exploitation—
May you live to say,
"Never again."

Contents

For Whom Is This Book Intended   xiii

Acknowledgments   xv

PART I.   *How to Become Assertive About Sex*   *1*

1   Taking Charge of Your Sexuality   **3**
Hazardous Recreation   *4*
The Risk to Men   *5*
The Risk to Women   *6*
What's in It for You?   *7*
What Is Sexual Assertiveness?   *9*
The Three Faces of Assertiveness   *12*
Verbal Self-Defense   *14*
Your Responsibility   *14*
Rewriting TV Lines: You're the Director   *14*

2   Learning the Basic Skills   **17**
Your Sexual Rights   *17*
The Payoff for Being Honest   *21*
Your Body Language and Tone of Voice   *22*
If It Ain't Broke, Don't Fix It   *23*
I-Statements   *23*
"How Dare You?"   *26*
Staying Sober   *26*
Using Your Own Words   *27*
Make an I-Statement   *27*
Sexual Ethics Checklist   *28*

3   Making Your Thoughts Work for You   31
Cultural Messages   32
Mind Versus Body   34
Family Scripts   35
Beliefs You Will Need   36
Common Beliefs about Sex   38
Beliefs About Your Health   39
Self-Esteem   40
How to Reward Yourself   40
Real Courage   42
Guided Imagery   43
Thought-Stopping   43
The Parts of You   44
Feeling Down   46
Self-Hypnosis   47
The Holistic Approach   48
Which Were You Scripted to Believe?   49

PART II.   *How to Respond to Persuasion*   51

4   Standing Up to Verbal Pressure   53
The Customs of Sexual Pressure   53
Using Your Higher Brain Power   55
Brainwashing   55
Recognizing Pressure Lines   56
Ideal Sexual Assertion   59
Your Policy Statement   60
Adults Can Be Abstinent   62
Vigilantes Out to Clean Up Sex Ed   64
Arousal and Guilt   67
Sharing a Partner   68
How Men Can Respond to Pressure   68
How Women Can Respond to Pressure   71
Your Body Is Not Debatable   73
How to Deal with Being Rejected   74
Talking about Your Sexual Policy   75
How Would You Answer?   76

5   Speaking Up to Avoid Disease and Pregnancy   79
How Widespread Are the STDs?   79
Finding Your Risk Triggers   83
Mother Nature's Plan   84

Three Basics about STDs   85
The First Conversation   87
Key Phrases to Remember   88
Explaining Ahead of Time   90
Mentioning Protection without Accusing   91
Imperfect Talk Is Okay   92
Lying Is Common   93
Getting Specific   93
How to Ask for a Condom   94
Other Condom Comebacks   96
Condom Realities   97
Asking for Birth Control   97
Discussing Your Outlook on Abortion   98
Time Out! What to Say in the Middle of Things   99
How to Ask for an STD Test   100
If You Have Exposed Someone to an STD   102
Legal Issues   102
Defend Yourself and Your Partner   103
How Would You Answer?   103
Is Alcohol a Risk Trigger for You?   104

PART III.   *How To Cope With Intrusion and Force*   107

6   **Resisting Sexual Harassment**   **109**
What Is Sexual Harassment?   109
What Is Not Harassment?   112
The Price Society Pays   113
The Stages of Sexual Harassment   114
Assertive Coping Skills in Dealing with the Harasser   114
Learning a New Professionalism   115
The Pressure to "Smooth It Over"   117
Getting Your Professionalism Across   117
How to Reward or Punish the Harasser   118
Resist Flattery   120
Folksy Little Maneuvers   121
When the Harasser Persists   121
Making a Joke   123
Avoid Being Alone with the Harasser   123
Keeping a Record   124
Arranging a Talk   124
Writing a Letter   125
Seeking Emotional Support   126
Other Options Before Taking Legal Action   126

Legal Remedies   127
Prevention of Further Harassment   127
If You Think You've Harassed Someone   127
Unethical "Helping" Professionals   128
Treatment for Sexual Harassers   130
Assertiveness on Tap   130
Construct a Conversation to Confront the Harasser   131

7   Avoiding Acquaintance Rape   133
Rape-Free Societies   134
The Culture of Rape   134
How Can Rape Be So Common?   137
How to Recognize a Potential Rapist   141
Talking to Rape-Prone Males   142
Rules for Avoiding Acquaintance Rape   145
Who Has Successfully Repelled Attempted Rape?   147
How Some Men Justify Rape   149
What Men Can Do to Prevent Rape   150
If You've Been Sexually Abused   152
If You've Been Raped   152
To Avoid Attempted Stranger Rape   153
For Help Immediately After a Rape   153
Legal Options   154
Treatment for People Who Use Sexual Force   154
Survivors Can Heal   154
Powell's Picnic   155

8   Responding to Other Intrusions   159
Persuading, Intruding, and Coercing   159
Degrees of Sexual Intrusion and Coercion   160
Uninvited Sexual Staring   162
Uninvited Sexual Comments   165
What to Say to Uninvited Sexual Comments   167
Obscene Phone Calls   168
Exhibitionists and Voyeurs   170
Protecting Yourself from Stalkers   171
Which Intrusions Have You Experienced?   173

PART IV.   *How To Speak Up For Your Society*   175

9   Searching for the Causes   177
Whatever Happened to Moral Outrage?   177

Can the Media Cause Sexual Violence? 178
Censorship and the Rape Culture 179
The Findings of Government Commissions 180
The Humor-Aggression Connection 180
Desensitization 182
Watching Sex without Aggression 183
The New Media Nymphomaniacs 185
Watching Aggression without Sex 186
The Catastrophic Linking of Sex and Aggression 187
The Problem with Macho 191
Females Who Encourage Macho in Men 192
Facing the Truth 192
When Is it Okay to Portray Sex or Violence? 193
Rating Your Favorite Movies and TV Programs 194
Sexual Messages in the Media 194
Aggressive Incidents in the Media 195

10 Becoming a Witness 199
Where to Begin 200
How to Speak Up in Social and Business Situations 201
Challenge the Myths 203
When You See Movies or Programs with Others 203
But I Can't Talk Like That 204
Other Chances to Respond 205
Insist on Fairness to Men 206
Make Phone Calls 206
How to Refer Someone for Help 206
Speaking Up to the Media 207
Boycott All Products that Involve Sexual Exploitation 207
Call or Write Letters 208
*Thank the Media that Present Entertainment Containing No Sexual
    Exploitation* 208
Demonstrate or Picket 208
How to Pressure Others to Change the Media 209
Ask for Prebriefings and Debriefings 211
Where to Ask for These Changes 212
Speaking Up for Children 213
Support Involved Fathers 215
Insist on Education 216
Be of Good Courage 217
If You Add Your Voice 217
Debrief Your Friends After the Movie 217
Respond to These Jokes 218

Appendix: Where to Get and Give Help   221

Preventing Sexual Aggression in the Media   221
Disease Prevention and Birth Control   223
Hotlines   223
Help for Children   225
Help for Violence at Home   225
Help for Alcohol and Drug Abuse   225
Help for Survivors of Sexual Exploitation   225
Your Personal Safety Checklist to Prevent Stranger Rape   226
Sources of Help for Sex Offenders   228
If You Need Psychotherapy   229
Research Data on Alcohol and Sexual Risk   229

For Whom Is This Book Intended?

As we move toward the turn of the century, sexual dilemmas may become increasingly difficult. Both men and women need skills to talk with other people about their sexual policies. Grappling with uncomfortable situations, they need the ability to speak up—to people they date, to bosses and co-workers, to professors and teachers, and sometimes even to unethical helping professionals or intrusive strangers. People need to know how to explain their opinions on becoming sexually involved, how to back someone off, and even how to avoid being falsely accused. If abstinence is their choice, they need the words to make that clear. Often knowing what to say in itself can result in more positive relationships and certainly in a greater sense of control over the major sexual issues of our lives. Coping with awkward, delicate, or perplexing situations in many cases boils down to, "What could I say—to make sure that my sexual choices take place on my own terms?" Over the years, as a psychologist, I have had students and clients, and others from fifteen to fifty, share their sexual dilemmas with me. Their struggles to find their own voices inspired me to write this book.

I will use *he* or *she* interchangeably throughout the book in the interest of helping all readers to relate to the examples. All the examples in this book (except those related to pregnancy) can apply equally well to people of either gender and any sexual orientation. If anecdotes involve real people, their names have been changed. In considering what to say or do in any sexual dilemma, you may use this book to help you find options. But ultimately you must then use your own judgment about which options to attempt.

Although this book contains information about legal and medical issues, that information is not intended as legal or medical advice. To locate an attorney for advice on a specific matter, contact your local bar association or lawyers' reference service for a list of licensed attorneys who practice in the area of your concern. To locate a physician, contact your local medical association. This book also suggests resources for readers seeking help. Many of these are national organizations with local affiliates, which may vary in the actual services and the quality of the services provided.

Acknowledgments

I would like to thank the following people for their patient evaluation and criticism: Mary Angelides, Joseph Dunne, Lee Ehrenberg, Barbara Fine, Peter Griffin, Shari Klein, Barry Schapiro, Sharon Burton Smith, Byron Walker, and Susan Waugh. I am grateful to Meg Selig, Joan Hartmann, and Margaret Terry for brainstorming. I am also indebted to Robert Gillespie for advice on biological matters. Melinda Smith, Rayna Morrison, and Michele Smith are much appreciated for criticisms from the single's viewpoint. I owe special thanks to Amy Salniker for her most pertinent comments. I also want to thank Lois Vander Waerdt for her advice on legal issues. And if it were not for Ellen R. Green Wood and Samuel E. Wood, authors whose enthusiasm brought this book to the attention of Allyn and Bacon, I might not have a publisher with whom I'm so pleased to work.

In addition, the comments of the following reviewers have been most helpful: Beverly Drinnin, Des Moines Area Community College; Susan Ann Lyman, University of Southwestern Louisiana; and Jan Francis, Santa Rosa Community College.

I am grateful to my students for sharing their questions and concerns—particularly the role players, whose courage helped me see what skills are needed for sexual safety.

And lastly, I honor the tradition of my Kentucky mountain kinfolk from the past and present, people of profound integrity and kindness. I especially cherish the steadfast example of my mother and father, who showed me that it is always possible to treat people right.

Sex on Your Terms

Part I

How To Become Assertive About Sex

1

Taking Charge of Your Sexuality

If I am not for myself, who will be for me? If I am only for myself, what am I?—And if not now, when?—HILLEL

Never before has a society provided so many ways to get into sexual trouble. Our country has the highest teenage pregnancy rate in the industrialized world. Five sexually transmitted diseases have reached epidemic proportions; the most serious of these—Acquired Immune Deficiency Syndrome, or AIDS—has caused thousands of deaths, and the virus has infected hundreds of thousands more who do not yet show symptoms.[1] The United States has one of the highest rates of rape in the world: At least one in four American women will be raped in her lifetime and many more will experience sexual assaults that do not result in completed rapes. Gay bashing—physical attacks on men believed to be gay—have caused an increasing proportion of men to be admitted to emergency rooms in recent years. Sexual dysfunctions and even total lack of sexual desire are becoming distressingly common among both males and females. Our children are not sexually safe, sometimes even from their own parents and often from others in whose care they have been placed. One of seven boys and one of four girls is sexually abused before the age of puberty.[2] In short, our country is a sexual disaster area.

Even more remarkable in the face of all these sexual problems, the majority of our citizens consider themselves incapable of, or unwilling to, talk about the very subjects that could drastically reduce or prevent many of these problems. Thousands could die and millions more become infected with a deadly disease that is sexually transmitted, but our society is so sexually impaired that many of its

3

politicians, educators, and religious leaders would not so much as mention the kind of protection that might save those lives.

Hazardous Recreation

The media overwhelm us with a barrage of sexual innuendos, titillation, and jokes, yet leave us without training or knowledge or permission to talk about sexual subjects in a healthy, assertive way. The typical American owns a little electric picture box that runs an average of seven hours a day,[3] and it portrays some of the most manipulative sex to be found anywhere. Not only is rape between lovers portrayed in the soaps on a regular basis,[4] but a recent survey found that over 60 percent of the music videos played on TV contained at least one of the following: degrading sexual portrayals, sexually suggestive themes, explicit violence, suggestions of violence.[5] We shall see how, even without sex, violent images contribute to sexual victimization.

Print media are equally likely to highlight unhealthy sex. Popular novels overflow with themes of unsafe, casual sex or sex that treats women as objects. Marty Klein, a noted sex educator, describes how the typical American romance novel involves a rape:

> *She's lonely, she's bored, she's cranky . . . and then some handsome stranger arrives in town. He looks her over but at first, she's not interested. There's coercive sex. During the coercive sex she has a revelation that he desires her so much he is willing to do this terrible thing of breaking the conventional morality and actually raping—or forcing her—and she comes to look at him in a new light. . . . She pursues him for the next couple of hundred pages. He is cold. He is aloof. But finally he comes to realize that Yes. . . . He does love her. And then they have a totally different kind of sex in the last 100 pages— . . . this sweet, romantic, bonding, intimate experience. . . .* [6]

Not only do females learn dangerous sexual attitudes from what's in print, but also young adolescent males cut their teeth on sexual violence. When they should be learning how to treat a woman with respect, they can easily obtain magazines depicting nude women being strung up and tortured. Or they can see slasher films in which sexy women are raped, stalked, or killed. Sex is becoming so linked with violence that an issue of *New York* magazine depicted a collar of nails on the cover, overlaid with the message "In 1974, It Was Free Sex. In 1984, It Was Safe Sex. In 1994, It's . . . Mean Sex."[7]

Unhealthy sex is all around us, flagrantly used to capture our attention and our money. But examples of healthy sex are harder to get than an X-rated film. If we had been born into a peace-loving, respectful tribe, much of this would not be so.

We would not be barraged by constant sexual messages that contradict the healthy messages we need. We would not have to find ways to protect ourselves sexually, because very likely no one would attempt to violate our sexual rights. Community standards and group disapproval would squelch an aggressive impulse before it became an action. We still might need to know how to talk about sexual matters, however, either to ask for something we need, to explain something sexual to some-one, or to refuse an undesired partner.

The Risk to Men

Men may doubt that they need to know how to deflect sexual pressure—it's not their problem. But both men and women need the skills to talk about sex in a vari-ety of situations. The good news is, if men learn to communicate better, they can enhance not only their relationships but also their work lives. Contrary to popular belief, men are sexually pressured by both male and female employers. Fifteen per-cent of the males in the federal work force claim to have been sexually harassed on the job.[8] Even if this number is an exaggeration, as some experts claim, men need to learn the facts about sexual harassment.

Males suffer, too, for other men who really are bad guys. Their high rate of sex-ual crimes against women makes even innocent men appear dangerous, and this fear is exaggerated in the way they are often depicted as sex-driven madmen in the media. Men in this society never know when they are going to be falsely accused of a sexual mistake. Some of my male colleagues (teachers, therapists, and other professionals) are more than a little jittery about the possibility that someone might fabricate a charge against them. What if they are affectionate, and accidentally pat a woman on the back or the hand in an effort to reassure her? Victims of sexual harassment have become more successful in the courts; does this mean that inno-cent men will be prosecuted? Knowing some simple ways to cope with these issues will help you to steer clear of on-the-job behaviors that could derail your career.

Men are at risk for sexually transmitted diseases; heterosexual intercourse is the fastest growing category for transmitting the virus that causes AIDS.[9] And without negotiating how to protect themselves or their partner, they can impreg-nate someone with whom they never would have had sex if they had been think-ing rationally. Often, gay men and lesbians are equally deficient in the skills need-ed for sexual safety.

Less visible but widespread is the fact that in our current climate, men simply are not trusted very much by the average woman looking for a partner. Even the most lovable and respectful man can be suspect to the woman who is struggling with memories of other men who were not so nice. How many men feel uncom-fortable when, walking behind a woman at night, they notice her speeding up and realize she is afraid of them? When their daughters, their sisters, their wives, and the women with whom they are involved have been victimized, men also pay a price. What another has done to the woman a man loves may haunt her and change how she relates to him.

Our national fascination with the dominant, rough man confuses women's attitudes and distorts their choice of men. One of my students asked, "Do nice guys finish last?" An article in a recent *New Woman* poses the puzzling question, "Are Nice Guys Boring in Bed?"[10] If nice guys are boring, whom does that leave to be interesting in bed, and how good can a relationship be with such a man?

Males are hurt by the problems of living in a society that refuses to deal with sexual matters in a straightforward way. And even the perpetrators of sex crimes are victims. They are damaged by our resistance to coping with sex, for in their histories there are invariably critical moments when sexual assertion could have helped. Many abusers, rapists, exhibitionists, and obscene phone callers have been victimized in some way in childhood, often in their own families. Professionals dealing with such families just don't hear them talk about sexual assertiveness and respect for sexual rights. A society that took sexual assertiveness for granted might have prevented the chain of abuse.

The Risk to Women

Although men can be exploited sexually, women have been the main victims of sexual exploitation for centuries. My own great-grandmother, to whom this book is dedicated, was a typical example. After the Civil War, when her family's tiny Virginia farm was looted, she went at age fourteen to work on a plantation in Tennessee. There she was sexually harassed, raped, and impregnated by the plantation owner. That man was my great-grandfather. Granny later married another man and brought her son over the Cumberland Gap into Kentucky, where our family has lived for over a hundred years. When I knew her, she was a little, stooped woman in a mountain bonnet who lived to be ninety-six. I would never have heard her story except for the fact that my uncle—the youngest of my great-grandmother's twelve grandchildren and a historian—revealed it to me during a visit a few years ago. Granny's story is a common example of the price women have had to pay for their lack of power. Assertion might have helped, but usually victims are unable to resist.

To a great extent, powerless people are the chief victims today. In *Human Sexuality*, Masters and Johnson, our foremost sex therapists, say, We live in a society that trains and encourages females to be victims of sexual coercion and males to victimize females.[11] That training comes by way of the message absorbed by American males—don't be assertive, be aggressive, be dominant. Our expectations of men are described by one expert in sexual violence:[12]

Masculinity in our culture includes independence (from relationships), lack of sentimentality, sexual success, . . . physical toughness, and worldly success, measured in dollars or achievements. Each of these elements of constructed masculinity has implications for a male's relationships with women. . . . Attachment to a woman can threaten the image of independence and produce accusations that a man is "dominated" or "pussy-whipped" by his mother, girlfriend, or wife.

Young teenagers learn to look at girls as pawns in a game. Two male professionals in the rape prevention field describe the aggressive sex language that many men use—" . . . I *porked* her, *stuck* it to her, *ripped off* a piece of ass"—as a means of making a woman into an object, a non-person.[13]

And the message we offer to females: Don't be assertive, be passive; you won't be loved if you aren't nice. This kind of background distorts the behavior of a typical couple, making the man aggressive and the woman uncomfortable about being assertive—a combination that is dangerous because it often ends in sexual abuse.

And so the man typically does not communicate in words, since he is trained to be silent and compete for all the sex he can get ("score"). He is taught to be emotionless, tough, and ready to fight—qualities that are quite helpful if he's flying a bombing mission over a foreign country, but disastrous in a human relationship. If he isn't really this tough, he hides it from other men and is afraid to show his sensitive side to women.

Because we don't know what to say, or are afraid to say it, we accept these affronts to our humanity. We need to stop the silence that results in nonassertiveness and sexual harm. We must make sure everyone knows how to talk about sexual concerns, just as we teach people how to drive safely. What was good enough for the forties is not good enough for the exploitative twenty-first century.

What's in It for You?

If you can be sexually assertive, you can enhance your sexual relationships and protect yourself in a variety of ways. If you have chosen to be abstinent, you can also explain your policy in more assertive terms and be more comfortable with it. In particular, if you are assertive you can:

1. *Decrease, or completely eliminate, your risk of contracting a sexually transmitted disease (STD).* Asserting your needs for information and protection is a basic necessity and responsibility if you are sexually active and are not in a longstanding, faithful relationship. Except in a case of rape, you largely control your exposure to STDs.

2. *Decrease your risk of pregnancy or of impregnating someone.* The rate of unwanted pregnancy in nonassertive individuals is far higher than in those who ask for protection. Two-thirds of sexually active American teenagers do not use contraception during their first act of intercourse. When asked why, they often report that they could not speak of such things. Many have intercourse when they don't even feel ready, but can't assert themselves enough to refuse. Well-meaning adults may tell them to just say no, but they don't know how. Yet many of them can easily use the most graphic sexual words to insult each other.

3. *Decrease your odds of being raped by an acquaintance, or of being accused of rape.* I want to be very careful not to suggest that all sexual victimization could have been avoided or is in some way caused by unassertiveness in the victim. Any rape is always the responsibility of the perpetrator, and often the victim could have done nothing to prevent the rape, or else could think of nothing to do under such stress. But when rape is on the mind of an acquaintance, the potential victim's assertiveness can sometimes change the balance of power. This effect is important because rape is primarily a crime of anger and power. A rapist's fantasies of a passive partner who says No when she means Yes are more likely to be discouraged by an assertive attitude in the intended victim. This is why I include the possibility of learning to use assertiveness in certain sexual situations before coercion can happen.

Moreover, a male who does not understand the politics of rape in this country often rapes a woman and does not even know he has committed a crime. A major national study found that one in every twelve men admits to committing acts that meet the legal definitions of rape or attempted rape.[14] If he forces intercourse on his date, perhaps when they have had a few drinks, he may not know it is a felony—because he thinks rape only comes from strangers. There are college men in prison for this misunderstanding.

4. *Decrease the odds of being sexually harassed, or of being accused of harassment.* Sexual harassment is sexual pressure from someone who has power over you in some way, such as your teacher or employer. Chapter 6 will explain more precisely what constitutes harassment. As with acquaintance rape, an assertive student or employee may not be as easy to harass as a nonassertive person. As more and more people know how to assert their sexual rights, others may be more reluctant to intrude upon these rights. Furthermore, understanding what constitutes sexual harassment will do much to prevent you from unknowingly engaging in this illegal act.

5. *Help yourself in other ways, such as knowing what to say to influence what is happening in your society.* Or you may wonder how to handle unusual situations, such as obscene phone calls or exposure to an exhibitionist; should you say anything to sex offenders you encounter?

The French refer to it as "the staircase phenomenon"—thinking of what you should have said as you are going back down the stairs after the opportunity has been lost. As you learn sexual assertiveness skills, you will find fewer and fewer regrets over what you might have said. I have an intense faith in the power of words. Although words cannot accomplish everything, it is often remarkable what saying the right thing can do. I have often asked myself where my intense belief in the power of our voices originated. Once, as a young child, I was locked in a trunk while playing and nearly suffocated. Although I had already learned to be the sweet, quiet little girl that my community expected of me, I pounded on the inside of that trunk lid and screamed for my mother with every ounce of my strength. She came quickly, and I was safe. When I ponder why my entire career has been based on what to say, I believe that first, profound lesson somehow imprinted upon me the power of my voice. Your adult voice can have power. Learn to use it well.

Most of us have come from families that discouraged us from speaking up about precisely what we need or feel. Well-meaning parents could not possibly have foreseen how necessary sexual assertion would be to their children's welfare. They usually were not taught assertion. They met fewer strangers; mutual trust and concern about reputation ensured their sexual safety in most situations. Our society previously depended upon the good manners of each person and rewarded humility and reticence; children learned to avoid a "big head" or a "smart mouth." Those who misused their power by harassing, abusing, or raping were not, as a rule, discovered or discussed. Like my great-grandmother, the victims were powerless.

Over the last fifteen years I've asked my students to write about how they deal with their anger. Their answers are a startling product of our culture. They believe anger must either be held in—which they see as harmful—or let out in a destructive way, such as in tantrums or violence. And some people feel this way about sex—that there are only passive and forceful choices available. It is remarkable how few of them realize that there are other options between these two extremes.

What Is Sexual Assertiveness?

No one likes a pushy person. You would not want to be so intent on your own rights that you become rude or trample on the rights of well-meaning people. One reason more of us are not able to assert ourselves is positive, in a sense: We are trying to avoid angry or rude outbursts and are afraid our anger will get out of control. Not knowing any halfway point between nonassertiveness and aggression, we keep quiet. Our assumption is that if we are not passive, we are aggressive.

Assertion, or *assertiveness,* is behavior in which you stand up for your rights and say directly what you believe, want, and feel. Assertive people do this appropriately and honestly while respecting other people's rights as well. The assertive person speaks up in her own defense, but does so without any effort to harm or put down another person. Let's listen to Tanika, who has been out with Derek several times. She's worried about sexually transmitted diseases, and their relationship has been getting more passionate. One night, after some kissing and petting that they both enjoyed, she decides to bring up her concerns.

Tanika: (Pushes Derek back and looks at him.) Derek. (Sigh.) I need to stop for a minute. I need to talk.

Derek: What for?

Tanika: Things are going pretty fast here, and I'm . . . just worried about going too fast.

Derek: What's to worry about if you feel good? (He tries to kiss her on the neck.) Come on, Tanny.

Tanika: (Leans back a bit.) Derek, you know I like you and I'm very attracted to you, but (she takes a deep breath) I think we need to talk before we go any further.

Tanika sticks to the point of what she needs. She expresses her views without putting Derek down. Since Derek was not out of line in merely wanting to continue enjoying what they were doing, she does not get angry.

Aggression, on the other hand, is behavior aimed at hurting or dominating. For example, consider Miguel and Kathy. They've been out a few times, and Miguel has asked Kathy to spend the night at his place.

Miguel: I wish you would, Kathy. You know how much I want to be with you.

Kathy: Cut it out, Miguel! You men are all the same!

Kathy's response is aggressive. She lashes out at Miguel and labels him and all men. Since Miguel was not manipulating her or using any force or coercion, she might really prefer that her outburst not escalate into bad feelings between them. She would rather have spared his feelings, since he was just asking for—not forcing—what he wanted. But she wanted to postpone further sex and she didn't know how to be assertive. An assertive response would have been:

Kathy: I know you want to, Miguel. But I'm just not ready for that yet.

Here she showed she was sensitive to his feelings, but she made clear what she wanted.

In a *nonassertive* response a person does not stand up for his or her own wants and needs. This behavior usually comes from feeling helpless and threatened. An example is Maria and Jim, who are sitting in the car, kissing. Maria starts to unbuckle Jim's belt. Jim takes her hand away.

Maria: Come on, Jim. You know I want you.

Jim: Oh, Maria, I don't know, I just . . . I don't think we should.

Maria: Just stay out here a little longer.

Jim: But, Maria . . . you know, you really turn me on, you know you do . . . but we just met last week and . . .

Maria: What kind of man are you? Am I ugly or something?

Jim: No, you're not. (She gives him a very long kiss.)

He's aroused and worries that he'll seem like a wimp if he says no. After a while they go inside and have intercourse, without a condom.

Jim did not stand up for his rights. Although he was aroused, he also was worried because he knew he was risking pregnancy and possibly disease if he rushed into sex with Maria. He allowed their arousal to progress to the point where he thought it was too late to discuss risk. And of course, as the old brain gets caught up in passion, Maria seems more and more wonderful and problem-free. There's a saying that anybody looks good at two o'clock in the morning. But he's known her only a week and could not possibly have enough information to justify taking a sexual risk with her.

Books about assertiveness training always give scenarios about what people say when they're not being assertive. But many sexual situations involve few, if any, words. If any words were spoken, the typical nonassertive scenario would go like this:

A: God!

B: (Kisses A, rubs body against A.)

A: (Pulls B closer, then pulls away.)

B: What? (Kisses A's neck.)

A: No, I. . . .

B: Please, just . . .

A: I . . . I . . . (Lies down on car seat, pulling B down on top.)

Assertiveness training has become popular all over the country as a way to help Americans learn how to speak up for themselves in a nondefensive, rational way that is most likely to solve problems. You can find classes in assertiveness training in most colleges and other adult education courses. Students are trained to be assertive but not aggressive. Yet in very few of these books or classes is sex ever mentioned. It is really all-but-sexual assertiveness training. Most teachers prefer to skip a subject as controversial and emotional as sex, and many audiences are self-conscious hearing about it. Partly because we avoid crude or distasteful sexual remarks in the interest of being well-mannered and polite, we make the entire subject taboo. Professionals sometimes feel embarrassed to treat the subject with their students or clients because they themselves are not at ease discussing such matters. Studies of physicians indicate a widespread inability to discuss sex with their patients. In a polite society, we implicitly agree not to discuss sexual matters. (If I say at a dinner party that I specialize in sexual assertion, an awkward silence follows.) Despite this great silence on the subject, I believe that sexual assertiveness is teachable. You may not be totally comfortable discussing sexual matters. That's normal in that most Americans feel such discomfort. But you deserve better.

Somehow, while growing up, I realized the absurdity of powerful adults—these people who knew all the answers—being reduced to embarrassed silence by the mere mention of sex. I hope you, too, see the insanity of allowing a taboo to threaten our society. Twenty years from now, our children will not thank us for saving them from hearing sexual words at the expense of their happiness and perhaps their lives.

Remember, assertion is just a tool to have in your repertoire. It is not a knee-jerk response to every situation. An example of a situation in which assertiveness was *in*appropriate involved one of my students, when a man phoned her, pretending to be taking a survey. As he started to steer the survey to sexual matters, she began to realize he was an obscene caller. She decided to say something assertive and retorted, "I'm getting very uncomfortable with these questions." Because she had thought she was dealing with a person who had some desire to be civil, she was using an assertive response instead of just hanging up. It was confusing for her. But some people need to be rejected outright. Some people are not only unworthy of your polite response but may also be dangerous. There will be times when you need to respond with a basic, primitive, protective reaction. No book can teach you that. But the purpose of this book is to teach you a set of assertive skills that you are unlikely to learn anywhere else. You need to have them available, but you do not have to use them in every situation.

The Three Faces of Assertiveness

Patricia Jakubowski and Arthur J. Lange, two of the best-known authors on the subject of assertiveness training, describe three kinds of assertion. These apply very well to sexual situations. The first kind of assertion is *empathic assertion*. In this case, you would assert yourself by first acknowledging the other person's feelings—that is, showing sensitivity to the other person.

For example, if Pat is being pressured verbally by Chris, Pat could be assertive and still empathic:

Chris: (Pulls Pat forward, kisses Pat.) Come on, Pat, please, what's holding us back?

Pat: I know you'd like to make love, Chris, but I'm not ready for that.

Here Pat has been self-respecting, but has been sensitive and does not try to hurt Chris. Pat sticks to the subject of personal reactions.

The second kind is *escalating assertion,* where you begin with mildly expressing yourself but, because your partner does not listen or respond, the intensity of your statements escalates:

Chris: Come on, Pat, you know you want me.

Pat: I . . . I'm just not ready to go that fast. Let's be responsible, like they say.

Chris: Come on, don't you want me? Pat, your body is just so . . . (Tries to pull Pat closer.)

Pat: I want you, too, but . . . not yet.

Chris: What's your problem? You got a problem with sex or something?

Pat: I really get mad when you talk like that! I said what I want to do, and I don't appreciate you putting me down.

Suppose Pat was a man. Does it seem strange to hear the man defending his right to refuse sex? Men of all ages are going to need to acquire the skills to be able to do this—and soon—if they are to protect themselves. And threatening a man's masculinity when he refuses sex is not an insult that men must disprove.

The third kind of assertion is *confrontive assertion.* You confront people who *do* something that contradicts what they *say.* Suppose, for example, Jason and Becky have a sexual relationship and have discussed using condoms. They've agreed that they will not have intercourse without one. Jason agreed to be responsible for buying them and Becky agreed to split the cost with him. One evening they begin to get sexually aroused and Jason clearly wants to have intercourse, but when Becky asks him, he does not have a condom. This is the third time this has happened. Becky confronts him.

Jason: Come on, hon, just this once won't matter. You can't get pregnant at this time of the month.

Becky: No, I told you how I feel. And people can get pregnant any time.

Jason: Hey, don't make a big deal.

Becky: I am really upset! You promised you'd take care of this and now you're trying to get me to take a risk because you forgot!

Here Becky confronts Jason directly with the fact that he has let her down and not kept his agreement. She doesn't let him get by with it, but because she thinks there is hope for this relationship she does not respond aggressively. She sticks to the point. She may be aroused, but she has not forgotten her own safety.

This book is intended to help the reader think of ways to say whatever needs to be said about sex—directly, honestly, and appropriately. These phrases don't usually come naturally. Every day, just by going to the movies or turning on the television, we can hear people saying things about sex that are devious, insulting, or manipulative. We have less experience seeing and hearing people discuss it in a healthy way.

Verbal Self-Defense

We spend a lot of time and money in karate and other kinds of self-defense classes. In one sense, this book is about self-defense training. But it is about verbal, not physical, self-defense. The characters in the scenes are responding to the words or actions of others, but only with words. Assertive language might help to prevent someone's using physical force against you; it might even stop someone in the midst of being violent. But once force is being used, there is physical risk, so other kinds of advice might be needed. Assertive responses are most effective when the person to whom you are speaking is capable of some rational thought. Please remember that this book refers only to prevention before physical force occurs. (For sources of help against sexual violence, see Appendix.)

Your Responsibility

No one can foresee the precise circumstances in which you may find yourself. Some potential sex offenders are dangerous. I hope you use this advice to increase your options, but ultimately you must rely on your own judgment as to which options you decide to attempt.

Rewriting TV Lines: You're the Director

Watch a television sitcom, a series, or a soap. Using the media checklists on pages 194–196 for guidance, choose one unassertive or aggressive comment made by any character. Rewrite the lines of that one character, but this time try to change the lines into a more assertive statement.

    1. Character actually said: _____.

    2. An assertive remark for that character would be _____.

NOTE: Did this changed line seem silly or awkward? Why do you think so? Why do you think assertive remarks in the media may seem out of place?

Notes

1. Centers for Disease Control National Hotline, January 16, 1995.

2. As cited by Thomas Lickona in *Educating for Character* (New York: Bantam Books, 1991), 351.

3. "A Little Less Time for TV," *U.S. News and World Report*, 19 June 1989, 74.

4. "Tune In Tomorrow," *St. Louis Post-Dispatch*, 8 January 1995, Sec. C.

5. Carole Lieberman, ed., *NCTV News* 13, nos. 2–4 (January–April, 1992), 1.

6. *Contemporary Sexuality*, 26, no. 7 (July 1992), 2–3.

7. *New York* 28 November 1994, 17, no. 47.

8. United States Merit Systems Protection Board, *Sexual Harassment in the Federal Workplace: Is it a Problem?* (Washington, D.C.: Government Printing Office, 1981) and U.S. Merit Systems Protection Board, *Sexual Harassment of Federal Workers: An Update* (Washington, D.C.: Government Printing Office, 1987).

9. Centers for Disease Control Hotline, December 16, 1994.

10. *New Woman*, December 1994.

11. William H. Masters, Virginia E. Johnson, and Robert C. Kolodny, *Human Sexuality* (New York: Little-Brown, 1991), 469.

12. Chris O'Sullivan, "Fraternities and the Rape Culture," in Emilie Buchwald, Pamela R. Fletcher, and Martha Roth, eds., *Transforming a Rape Culture* (Minneapolis: Milkweed Editions, 1993), 27.

13. Joseph Weinberg and Michael Biernbaum, "Conversations of Consent: Sexual Intimacy Without Sexual Assault," in Buchwald, Fletcher, and Roth, eds., *Trnasforming a Rape Culture*, 97.

14. Robin Warshaw, *I Never Called it Rape* (New York: Harper and Row, 1988).

15. Patricia Jakubowski and Arthur J. Lange, *The Assertive Option* (Champaign, Ill.: Research Press, 1978), 161–64.

2

Learning the
Basic Skills

> *I am not in this world to live up to your expectations, and
> you are not in this world to live up to mine.*[1]
> —FRITZ PERLS

Your Sexual Rights

Some people think they have no right to *ask* for what they want. Others feel they
do not have a right to *refuse* except under certain circumstances, sometimes even
in marriage. Some even believe that being made fun of in sexual ways at work,
while slightly embarrassing, is something they just have to endure. They wouldn't
feel so helpless if they were able to understand, and to state explicitly, their sexual
rights. Only then can they assert their power over their own bodies.

These fundamental rights, to which I believe everyone is entitled, are not all
legal rights, although some of them are built into our laws. You may want to add to
this list with ideas of your own.

1. *A person has a right to refuse any type of sexual contact at any time or place,
regardless of how aroused the partners might be.* There is no such thing as being
so aroused that you owe anything to your partner. If you are stark naked and change
your mind, you still have a *right* to do so. Now, if you take off your clothes and
change your mind on numerous occasions, you still have a right to do so, but there
is an element of game playing—and probably anger and manipulation—in it. It's
best if your body language agrees with what you're willing to do. Your body is still
yours, though, and you are the only one who can make decisions about it.

In my community college classes, students of all ages, role-play ways to resist sexual pressure. We set up four chairs and assume that the main couple is alone together. The other two chairs are for coaches who help out if the main players get stuck. Our role-plays do not involve touching; the audience has to imagine that. First the man verbally pressures the woman. Then they reverse roles and the man refuses the woman's pressure. Men are sometimes willing to participate in the first situation, but when the women pressure them, the younger men are invariably very tense and uneasy. Indeed, only a few brave ones volunteer for this exercise. They show such signs of anxiety as repeating phrases. They often cop out; instead of resisting pressure, they make up a reason why they cannot have sex: "I have a girl-friend already." Twice I've seen a male student sit down and refuse to play the role of a man turning down a woman. Some men are highly vulnerable in this society to the fear of appearing unmanly. Saying yes has been ingrained in them as the only position a real man can take. ("Go for it!" "Did you get any?") *This attitude must change,* or the rate of sexually transmitted disease (STD) will continue to increase at an alarming rate. Going out with someone, buying dinner, or doing other favors does not confer sexual rights to one person over another. This kind of misunder-standing, though, might be one good reason for women to start paying their own way or making the extent of their sexual availability clear before accepting gifts or favors. Unfortunately, some people are so confused that they feel they deserve something sexual for their money.

2. *A person has a right, in a sexual relationship, to express frustration and disappointment—in words—if sexual contact is refused.* If you refuse to continue some kind of sexual activity when both of you are very aroused, your partner has a right to express disappointment, respectfully. That is, other people have a right to their feelings, and you have a right to yours. However, a person who frequently asks for more sex and then expresses disappointment, even though the partner's position has been made clear, may be seen as a high-pressuring person. I knew a young, beautiful woman who asked her husband to make love at least once a day. He felt so pressured that he began to balk during lovemaking. Finally he let her know that he felt pressured, even though she asked with a big smile. Their sex life improved.

3. *A person has a right to any feeling, fantasy, or thought.* Whatever happens inside your head is yours. However, you are responsible for all of your behavior, which should not interfere with anyone else's rights. Normal people invent the weirdest fantasies and thoughts. Most of us would never dare share them with anyone else, for fear of being thought crazy or bad. Studies of fantasies reveal that far more people think about unusual sexual behaviors than actually do them. Your right to any thought does not mean that your thoughts are all healthy for you or for others. If, for example, a person is obsessed by certain thoughts, she may need professional help. If a stepdaughter is constantly bothered by daring sexual thoughts about her mother's husband, these thoughts might cause her to take actions that could endanger her family relationships. She might need the help of a counselor (see

Appendix for resources). Or a person could be a sexual addict whose distorted thoughts trigger exhibitionism or child abuse. Many Americans have a religious background which has not always made clear the boundaries between thoughts and actions. But mental health professionals tend to minimize the importance of people's thoughts and fantasies unless they trigger harmful emotions or actions.

4. *A person has a right to know if a potential sex partner has a contagious disease of any kind, or could possibly have been exposed to one.* Did previous lovers exhibit any of the symptoms of sexually transmitted disease listed on pages 80–81? Did they engage in any high-risk experiences such as sex with multiple partners, or belong to high-risk groups such as prostitutes or people who have shared intravenous drug needles? A couple contemplating a penetrative sexual act are taking certain chances, but each person has a right to hear whatever the other knows about the risk. You have a right to information and you should ask assertive questions. Your right to know, however, does not guarantee that your partner will tell the truth. Current research indicates that from one-third to one-half of sexually active people say they would lie to another person in order to get sex.[2] Trusting someone you do not know well with your body is simply not smart.

5. *A person planning sexual intercourse has a right to know whether the partner is using a contraceptive or other protective device and any pertinent facts about it.* Condom users have a right to know whether the condom is latex (the most effective kind), whether it is new or five years old, whether it is treated with a spermicide, and whether it is being used correctly. A man has a right to know whether his partner missed her pill any day that month.

6. *Partners involved in a sexual relationship have a right to share expenses that in any way result from their sexual involvement.* Their mutual obligation may include sharing the cost of contraceptives and expenses resulting from pregnancy. Deception by one, however, might change the rights of the other.

7. *A person has a right to be free from becoming the object of unwanted sexual remarks or unwanted sexual gestures.* "Look at the knockers on that broad!" yelled down from a construction site, or a whistle from the street corner, is a form of sexual intrusion. However, anyone who sees a sexually attractive person has a right to feelings that do not result in offensive behavior.

8. *A person has a right to use the telephone without the intrusion of uninvited sexual remarks or sexual threats.* An obscene phone call is an expression of hostility, a violation of sexual privacy, and another form of sex without consent. It is also a crime. The overwhelming majority of women in the United States have experienced this form of sexual intrusion. We should be deeply concerned that this practice of anonymously frightening someone with sexual threats is so widespread.

9. *A person has a right to be free from physical contact of any kind unless he clearly indicates a desire for it.* Between strangers, this prohibition is very clear.

Touching another person's buttocks, breasts, or genitals without consent, for example, is illegal in most states. And the consensus that exists in our society forbidding more extreme force, such as rape, is rarely a point of disagreement. However, some acquaintance rapists claim that they misunderstood the women's intentions. They may believe that her no means yes. Novels, television and films, and songs encourage that idea.

10. *A person has a right in a relationship with a helping professional (such as a doctor, psychologist, attorney, psychiatrist, member of the clergy, or teacher) to be free from any sexual suggestions, advances, or pressures.* The needy person seeking help is particularly vulnerable to the rationalizations and whims of those in positions of power and status. Although the relationship with such a professional is unequal, it is based on trust. The codes of ethics of most helping professionals prohibit any sexual contact or dating, and these professionals are well aware of the ethical implications. Many believe that a therapist who has intercourse with a patient should be charged with statutory rape.

11. *A person has a right to attend school at any level without unwelcome sexual pressure from faculty, school employees, or students.* It is not fair to interfere with someone's studies by means of any unwelcome sexual conduct, and it is against the law. This includes a wide range of behaviors commonly thought of as jokes, such as pulling down another teenager's bathing trunks in swimming class or a teacher's making hostile comments about stupid blondes.

12. *A person has a right to work at his/her place of employment free of unwelcome sexual pressures from employers or co-workers.* Federal statutes protect men and women from sexual harassment, which ranges from undesired sexual remarks to the actual discharge of an employee for resisting sexual overtures. (If some readers cannot imagine men being threatened by a sexual offer, only imagine yourself being propositioned by an employer who is extremely unattractive or whose sexual orientation is not the same as yours.) On the job, employees should be judged only by job performance and not for granting or refusing sexual favors.

13. *A person has a right to wear the clothing of choice, providing it is within the law.* Absolutely nothing you can wear (or not wear) gives anybody any sexual rights over you. A common myth that women's clothes cause male behavior is completely without basis. However, if others frequently react to your clothing with sexual remarks or arousal, you must confront the reality that somebody thinks you are communicating a sexual message you did not intend. If Tiffany wears a T-shirt that says "Make Me An Offer," she is within her rights, but she needs to know that it may provoke a sexual reaction. If Mary's blouse is transparent, she may be safer if she can anticipate its effect on other people. Despite their reactions, however, no one has a right to violate Mary's sexual rights. Until informed otherwise, those who see through Mary's blouse or read Tiffany's shirt should assume that these are clothing styles and not requests for sexual activity. They are never requests to be raped. Another area where clothing rights are relevant occurs when some employers require uniforms. Employees occasionally have protested the requirement to wear a revealing or seductive uniform in the workplace.

14. *A child has a right to be protected from any contact or experience with an adult that is for the purpose of that adult's sexual arousal or satisfaction.* This restraint goes beyond the types of sexual contact that are illegal, such as rape or molestation. It also includes words or gestures that the adult finds arousing. Children are amazingly sensitive; when they are being exploited it is recorded on an unconscious level.

15. *A child has a right to know what will happen to his or her body at puberty and the implications of those changes.* At present very few states require sex education in the schools, and political pressure prevents many of those from frankly confronting important issues. Some school districts have actually passed down directives that the words *intercourse* and *condom* are not to be mentioned in school. Yet very thorough sex education reduces the rate of disease and pregnancy.

Should the following also be a right, or is it just a desirable situation that one can hardly expect?

16. *A person has a right to know the intentions of a partner before they have sexual intercourse.* If it means strictly recreation to one partner, and love to the other, does each partner have a right to know about these feelings? Or is it merely important information—be careful, but you must take your chances, since love cannot be guaranteed?

You may have thought of rights that you could add to this list, or revisions you would want to make. But the major point is that there are certain givens for fair-minded people.

Thinking about these rights and integrating them is very important to your ability to be sexually assertive. If you do not believe you have sexual rights, your actions will reflect your fears and uncertainties. It is still never, ever your fault if someone forces you to do anything sexual. But it helps if you have a strong awareness of the issues involved. If you are dealing with a person who can be backed off, the efforts you make to protect yourself will carry more conviction when you know your rights.

The Payoff for Being Honest

If you are going to have happy relationships in your life, you are going to have to be honest. In our country, in times past, more people had pride in their honesty. My grandfather (remember the son of the plantation owner?) was a simple mountain man who could not even write. When he spoke with other mountain people, they often added a phrase to show the other that they were sincere: "'Pon my word and honor." It seems strange to me to have to explain the meaning of those words, but they aren't heard much nowadays. Your word—what you said or promised—was a source of pride, and going against your word was a reason for embarrassment and humiliation, or dishonor. A small-businessman, for example, would be ashamed to go back on his word, and his reputation would suffer. But this pride in personal honor is no longer a part of our culture; it seems old-fashioned and antiquated to some. Today we even have people who have stolen millions of dollars teaching at major universities. We have authors who make money writing about how to rip off other people or how they embezzled money, or betrayed our country. We have people who have been involved in major scandals who throw themselves into the public view on talks shows. This climate in which the dishonest person is admired and paid money may confuse you but you need to keep your focus: Moral standards are the only hope for our country and the only hope for relationships. And this does not mean that someone has to have your religion in order to be moral; there are moral people all over the world, with a variety of beliefs about religion.

Theoretically, being honest should be reward enough for its own sake. You should take pride in your personal ethics. But you also gain something for being honest and lose something if you are not. You gain a greater chance of being cared for by other people. By *honest* I do not mean compulsively frank, spilling your guts over every thought or fantasy you've ever had. I mean fair, just, and open about anything you would want to know if you were in the other person's place. Therapists and health educators all agree that honesty promotes smooth relationships and helps people attain closeness and even serenity.

There is always hope for change in people who have built their lives on dishonesty. True, some people who have antisocial personality disorders do not ever feel guilty and will probably always manipulate and seek victims. But others have turned around and have much more pride in themselves. Alcoholics Anonymous gives us some hopeful examples; after becoming sober, thousands of people have apologized and tried to make up for dishonest actions of the past.

You may need to take a good hard look at how honest and just you are in your interactions with other people. Or, you may need to take a deep breath and think about the morals of that person to whom you're so overwhelmingly attractive. Has that person been truthful with you? Have you ever found that person lying to you? If so, were you offended and did your relationship go into a crisis? Or did you just lower your standards and accept this affront? Think about it.

Your Body Language and Tone of Voice

You convince another person that you really mean what you say not only with words but, sometimes unconsciously, with gesture and posture. You might be able to say the assertive words, but unless your body conveys your sincerity, the words will sound canned and false. Your body shows your intent to stand up for your rights. Most people generally can look someone right in the eye. If you are assertive you hold up your head rather than hang it down sheepishly.

You can say the same thing in a whiny, scared little voice or with the strength of conviction. At your assertive best, your voice is not timid and uncertain but strong enough to show that you mean what you say. But when you're discussing difficult sexual topics—especially if you're sexually aroused—it's natural to hem and haw a bit at first. You should congratulate yourself on even beginning to open up these important subjects. The more you realize you have the rights described above, the more your total appearance and voice convey that you really mean what you say.

Nobody who's sexually aroused with another person can avoid at least one mixed message. You may "not want to" with your brain while your body language shows that you really "want to." You may say what you think is best for you after you've just been kissing or petting passionately with someone. It should be understood that, if you are doing this, you are attracted to the person and part of you wants to go further. Or, to put it another way, your higher brain has considered intercourse and decided to refuse it, while other parts of your brain and body are trying to propel you forward into a delightful passion.

So you need to decide what you're communicating to the other person if you say you don't want intercourse but your body language conveys the opposite. It's usually best if you explain how far you want to go so that the other person receives a more consistent message:

"I love to kiss but I don't want to go any further."

"It's important to me to keep my clothes on—that's sort of my boundary line."

"I need to let you know how far I want to go, because I'm so attracted to you, you may not realize that I. . . . "

If It Ain't Broke, Don't Fix It

Talking about sex may be easier than you think. Not everything you want to say requires expert advice. Recently I asked students to submit questions about sexual communication. One student wrote, "How do I tell a nurse I've been hit in the genitals with a baseball?" This illustrates the common fallacy that experts necessarily know better than we do. I told him to tell the nurse, "I've been hit in the genitals with a baseball."

I-Statements

If you need something or are asserting your right to something, it is best to speak clearly and straightforwardly. Of all the feedback I've ever received on sexual communication, the I-statement is the one students rave about the most. The I-statement is a simple tool that includes your emotional reaction. These expressions not only say what you think, but they stress how you feel. Myung Hee and Yuan for example, have been dating for a year. Sometimes when they go to parties Myung Hee spends most of the time talking to other guys, even when Yuan doesn't know anyone there. Yuan feels embarrassed and uncomfortable standing around by himself. After she's done this at several parties, he decides to be open about it:

Yuan: Myung, I am really getting irritated standing around alone at these parties!

Myung Hee: Hey, what's the problem, I just want to have a good time.

Yuan: Well, I'm very uncomfortable spending a whole night in a bunch of strangers.

Here Yuan takes responsibility for his own reactions in an assertive manner. He labels what he feels. He does not blame himself or Myung Hee.

It may seem like a big risk to lay your feelings open in this way. It makes you vulnerable. But if you *can't* say how you feel, you are a lot more vulnerable to things that will happen *later* if you don't speak up. One of the biggest mistakes in communication is the You-statement, which usually blames the other person. It puts him on the defensive and is usually aggressive. How would this scene above have gone if Yuan had made a You-statement?

Yuan: Myung Hee, you are the rudest person I've ever met, leaving me and going off whenever we go to a party. You couldn't care much about *me*.

Myung Hee: You are so insecure! Why don't you just start talking to people?

Is Myung Hee more likely to see Yuan's viewpoint after this? Not likely. She even makes a You-statement back to him. When people accuse and blame us, we're likely to go straight into defending ourselves. But after hearing people tell us their feelings, we have a chance to stop and think about their reactions to what we are doing. Here's a comparison of some important sexual communications contrasting I-and You-statements:

I-Statement	*You-Statement*
I feel pressured.	You are pressuring me.
I need more time.	You're always rushing me.
I'm embarrassed.	You shouldn't say that (or do that).
I'm scared.	You're scaring me.
I'm disappointed.	You let me down again.
I'm not ready for that.	You are too pushy.
I need to talk about our lovemaking.	You keep putting me off.

I'm not comfortable having sex without a condom.	You aren't considering my feelings about condoms.
I don't feel aroused.	You're not turning me on.
I'm really confused when you say that.	You are a liar.

You can learn a little starter phrase to get yourself going in order to make an I-statement. First, think of what you really *feel.* You're often experiencing some emotion, like pride, thrill, anger, irritation, guilt, jealousy, embarrassment, disappointment, fear, or discomfort. Then plug the emotion into one of these sentences: "I feel . . . when you do that." (or): "I'm . . . "(mentioning the feeling).

This technique may seem canned and artificial at first, but you'll get used to it so that you can fit I-statements into your conversations more easily. "I'm uncomfortable" is my favorite all-purpose I-statement. It can be used in many situations without having to give reasons. You can say you're uncomfortable when you can't pinpoint your exact feelings, but you feel a need to speak up anyway:

A: Remaining a virgin is important to me.

B: Why?

A: It just is.

B: You must have some reason.

A: It's what I've decided.

B: But why? Sex is good for you. You need it.

A: Look, I'm uncomfortable with all this pressure.

Men often need some defense when that dreaded threat to their masculinity is used against them:

A: You think you're such a big man, but you won't go to bed with me?

B: I really get mad when you try to question my masculinity like that!

Practice making such statements about small issues. They can help you in non-sexual situations, even with your family: "I'd like you to help me with this." "I'm so proud of you." "I'm disappointed that you were late." These expressions are not magic, of course. They are simply an improvement over most people's communication. In the area of sex, they are usually a vast improvement. For the best outcome, however, you need a willing listener who has some concern about your feelings. In other situations, like the above conversation about virginity, you may still want to state your position clearly even if the other person is not a good listener. I-statements *increase your odds* of getting your feelings across successfully to another person. That's what this book is really about—increasing your odds of protection by sexual assertiveness.

"How Dare You?"

I-statements assume that the other person is capable of concern when you say how you're reacting. In the field of communication there is great emphasis on not responding aggressively. But there are also times to shock someone who is out of line. There are times when you don't want to dignify what someone else has done or you don't trust the person enough to reveal your own feelings in an I-statement. For example, I knew a 16-year-old who was raped by a student at her high school (she found out later he was an obscene phone caller in her neighborhood). The rape was not only traumatic at the time but additionally upsetting because of the police efforts to prove she was lying. She finally gave up and decided not to prosecute. Numb, terrified, but trying to get her life back on course, she went to a party of high school students in her neighborhood. A male student came up and said in a casual, intrusive tone, "I heard John D___ raped you, is that true?" There was no response to make this situation all right, or to make herself feel good, but she replied from the gut, "How dare you!" turned around, and walked off. There are times when "How dare you!" is appropriate.

Staying Sober

Sexual assertiveness depends on higher brain functions. That means that you need to have a clear head so you can think about the consequences of your behavior and defend yourself if necessary with words or actions. You cannot think clearly under the influence of a mood-altering chemical such as alcohol, cocaine, or marijuana. *The overwhelming majority of young women who become pregnant unintentionally, contract a sexually transmitted disease, or are raped by an acquaintance, are intoxicated at the time.* Men can be raped—usually by a male—and drug use increases the odds of this kind of victimization. As many as three-quarters of sex offenders, particularly rapists, had been drinking at the time of their crime. Even a couple of drinks can lower your inhibitions against doing things that are self-destructive.

Recent surveys indicate that college students are engaging in more binge drinking than ever before. Alcohol is seen as the oil that gets the social machinery going, the prop to help people over awkward moments, whatever their age. But if you really want to mature, concentrate on building your confidence so that you can have fun, dance, and feel comfortable socially without alcohol or other drugs.

Many readers of this book will be untreated chemical dependents, or care about someone who is. Please, inform yourselves by calling the National Council on

Alcohol and Drug Abuse or other numbers listed in the Appendix. Then attend meetings and find out where to start on the road to sobriety. There is more help now than ever before.

Using Your Own Words

In the following pages I will suggest many ways to talk about sex. It is best for you to take what you like and rephrase it in your own words. Getting across *your meaning* is what counts.

Make an I-Statement

If you were involved in the following scenarios you might need to make an I-statement. Rather than focusing on the other person's actions, here you might want the other person to know how you're feeling. Even if the scene does not seem to apply to you, fill in the blank with an I-statement. Remember, after you make the I-statement you can also tell other people what you want. I-statements can be the beginning of a conversation and don't have to stand alone.

1. You pass your friend Jon's fraternity house, where he's standing with his buddies. As you pass, you can hardly believe your ears, because some of the brothers are yelling out numbers to rate your body. ("Hey, that's a seven!") You don't think Jon called out anything, but later you see him on campus. You want to tell him how you reacted.

   "Jon, yesterday when I passed your house and those guys yelled out, I felt ＿＿＿ because ＿＿＿."

2. You were Jon in the scene above. You were uncomfortable with the guys yelling at your friend. Afterwards you decide not to just let it ride, but to say something to them. You say, "When you were yelling out at her like that, I felt ＿＿＿ because ＿＿＿."

3. You are at a summer party where a young woman is coming on to you very seductively. She leans her body against you and whispers that you could leave the party and go off with her. You're startled at this sudden come-on and, even though she's attractive, you back off suspiciously. She keeps following you around, asking, "Why not?" "What's wrong?" You say, "I am getting really ＿＿＿ (mention your emotion) and I want you to ＿＿＿."

4. (Do this one if you're a male or female; the professor is a male.) You like your English professor and he asks you to go out one night and have a drink to discuss your paper. Looking back, you realize he was being seductive, but now the professor is putting his arm around you in the booth, breathing down your neck, and asking you to go to someplace more private where you can get to know each other. You say, "I am feeling ＿＿＿ and I want you to ＿＿＿."

5. You've had one date with someone you really like. Back at school, some of the guys who saw you two out begin to pressure you to "tell all." "Hey, did you get any?" one says. "Come on, what was she like?" You try to change the subject. "Aw," says one, I bet you just couldn't do anything when you tried, huh?" You say, "Lay off it, guys, I am really getting ____ when you guys ____."

6. You've decided to wait until you're engaged to have sexual intercourse. A group of friends is sitting around talking about sex and you say how you feel. A couple of people begin to kid you about this, trying to make you feel like a child. They won't let up. Finally you've had it. You say, "I am really ____ when you ____."

Sexual Ethics Checklist

How ethical are your sexual behaviors? Answer True or False to the following:

M&F __ 1. I would tell a potential sex partner if I had been exposed to a sexually transmitted disease.

M&F __ 2. If I were in a steady dating relationship and had sexual intercourse with someone else one time only, I would still tell my steady about it.

M&F __ 3. If I heard that a single woman with whom I work was very upset over finding she was pregnant, I would refrain from telling any of my friends at work.

M&F __ 4. If I were dating a person who had told me clearly and emphatically that he/she did not want to have intercourse, and we both became intoxicated and the person agreed to have sex, I would go ahead.

F __ 5. If I were a female who was crazy about a guy I was dating, and unexpectedly had a chance to have intercourse with him, I would tell him I was on the pill even if I was not, knowing I'd get on it the next day for sure.

M __ 6. If I knew my male friend was very pushy with women, and he asked me to set it up to leave him alone with a female friend of mine who did not know him, I would refuse to participate.

M&F __ 7. If I was in a group that was laughing at a movie that made light of rape or a rape attempt, I would tell them I didn't like to see rape be made a joke of like that.

M&F __ 8. If my friends pressured me to brag about someone I had dated— whether we had done anything sexual or not—I would refuse to talk about private things between us.

F&M __ **9.** If I were sexually involved with someone and I did not believe in abortion as a choice, I wouldn't bring up the subject for fear that I might lose the other person.

M __**10.** If the guys had drilled a hole into the women's locker room wall and I knew the women being viewed would feel terribly violated if they knew, I would refuse to participate.

M&F __**11.** If a potential sex partner asked me what kinds of sexual risks I had taken in my life, I would tell the truth.

M&F__ **12.** If I were in the heat of passion with someone who was saying "No" and I thought of some line I could say to get the other person to go ahead, I probably would.

Now, what is your score? The most ethical answers would probably be *True* to 1, 2, 3, 6, 7, 8, 10, and 11; and *False* to 4, 5, 9, and 12.

But surprise! Your answers may not have much meaning. Why not? Because people tend to answer questions the way they think they *should* rather than responding the way they *would* in the real pressure situations of life. It sounds good to say we wouldn't do anything unethical. But it requires character to follow up. It requires a constant ability to put ourselves in another's place.

Notes

1. Frederick S. Perls, *Gestalt Therapy Verbatim* (Lafayette, Calif.: The Real People Press, 1969), 1–4.

2. David Wheeler, "College Students Put Sex Partners at Risk of AIDS by Lying About Past Experiences," *Chronicle of Higher Education* (21 March 1990); Daniel Goleman, "The Lies Men Tell Put Women in Danger of AIDS," *New York Times*, 14 August 1988.

3

Making Your Thoughts Work for You

> *. . . there are certain "silent assumptions" that probably still lurk in your mind.*[1]—*DAVID BURNS*

"I can't help it—I can't help myself." So ran Darryl's thoughts as he decided to have unprotected intercourse with his third partner that week. But nobody forced him to take that risk. In actuality, Darryl made a choice. Thousands of people take precautions against sexual risks, and they feel just as passionate as Darryl did. But there is a crucial difference between Darryl and those people: what they *believe*. Darryl believed he was helpless against his sexual impulses, so he did not try to protect himself or his partner.

Because she *believed* she would lose her boyfriend if she insisted on a condom, Jackie became pregnant. She is not unusual; in fact, even teens who have been sexually active for some time tend to use either unreliable methods or no birth control at all. Why? Because they believe they cannot get pregnant, or they feel it is unromantic, or they think that women should not be assertive.

The things you believe are the among the most powerful influences in your life. And the good news is that you can gain some control over these thoughts and ideas. The decisions people make depend upon what they believe. They are usually unaware of how their beliefs guide them, but these assumptions lie there in the background at every moment. If you strongly believe something, it's all you can do to keep that attitude to yourself. Can you pick out what Paul believes?

Angela: You're lucky I'm dating you—probably not many women would go with a guy who has your eye problem.

Paul: (Looking miserable.) I just know . . . I don't want to break up with you.

Paul has an eye problem that gives his eyes an unusual appearance. But why did Paul let Angela get by with such an insulting remark? *Because he really believes nobody else would care about him.* If he thought he had a right to be treated with respect, he could have told Angela how he feels about her remark.

Your beliefs show not only in what you *do* but also in your tone of voice, your facial expressions, even the pauses in your conversation. Regardless of whether you try to hide what you believe, your act will often have very little impact. It might even confuse the other person. Your sexual beliefs—about your rights, your ethics, your pleasures—are like a computer programmed to guide your actions. And this programming comes from a variety of outside sources.

Cultural Messages

Our society beams scores of sexual messages at your eyes and ears every week. Some are positive. A major shift during the last fifty years, for example, has popularized the concept that adults are sexual beings and that sexual feelings are a normal part of human life. But more often cultural messages confuse us and undermine our natural tendency to act in our own best interest. Whereas these societal messages are rarely written down, they are definitely implied.

See whether you notice anything peculiar about the following remarks:

She: Come on, Phil, what are you saving your virginity for?

He: I'm just not ready. (He lowers his eyes shyly.)

Lochiel took him in her arms with the strength of months of waiting, and felt him slowly begin to respond.

Maggi was the most powerful woman in the company, and when Jack saw her pass his desk he secretly dreamed of the day when she would speak to him.

Did any of these comments snag you? They probably did, because each reverses our cultural messages that tell men and women how they are supposed to act.

Male Messages

At a very early age, little boys pick up the message that it's a catastrophe to act like a sissy. Soon they get the point that they are supposed to compete to get sex from girls and, hopefully, become a real stud. Occasionally this goes as far as the Spur Posse in California, a teenage male club whose members were accused of raping girls to get points. It seems the Posse gave points only if it was a different female each time, so the members were under pressure to find cooperative females. But even when male attitudes do not reach this extreme, young men have fears of not being dominant. When a woman pressures a man, he often cringes from the role reversal because he believes he should stay in the powerful role. Everything in his society has taught him to believe this so-called fact.

The powerful role has one major requirement in sexual situations: A powerful man must conquer a woman sexually, certainly not submit to any of her requests. So when a woman insists that a man use a condom, the man's fear of giving in to a woman may cause him to refuse. Men even have words for dominated men: *pussy-whipped,* or *hen-pecked.* But this fear of losing control is dangerous to his health, and to hers. It contributes to the fact that one in every thirteen American women has been physically abused by a man.

You'd think that young males with traditional beliefs would be more reticent than other men about sex and women. But it looks as if some traditional beliefs can lead to dangerous behaviors. The National Survey of Adolescent Males recently studied over 600 young men from a variety of ethnic groups, including white males, and asked them if they held traditional attitudes like these:

I admire a guy who is totally sure of himself.
Men are always ready for sex.
I don't think a husband should have to do housework.
A guy will lose respect if he talks about his problems.

They found that the males who agreed with this kind of traditional statement were sexually at risk—and so were their partners. These young men had more sex partners in the last year, used condoms less consistently, and believed men were less responsible than women for preventing pregnancy than did men with nontraditional beliefs. What is even more alarming is that these young men believed that pregnancy proves a man's masculinity and that relationships between the sexes are based on rivalry and competition—that men and women are basically opponents.[2]

Female Messages

On the other hand, we do not encourage women to seek competition and power but instead to value love and relationships. And even when they do need to be powerful, women often do not realize they have that potential. Girls pick up the message that they are supposed to be nice and loving, and to wait until they are chosen. So a woman may be scared of losing the love of a man if she shows power by insisting on her sexual rights. In some minority communities, for example, it is unthinkable for a woman to insist on a man's doing anything—he cannot be macho if he gives in. Women need to learn new skills in order to insist upon condoms and other sexual protection. But they also need to *believe* that they can be feminine and still have power over themselves.

Beliefs about male and female roles are just a few of the sexual beliefs stored there in your mind, guiding you all the time. But if you're going to protect yourself, you're going to have to think rationally, in an unclouded way. You can't act in your own interest if your beliefs are confusing you.

Take my student, Jean, for example. We were role-playing with Mark, who was doing a great job carrying out his instructions to be pushy. Jean, who was instructed to assert herself, seemed uncomfortable. Their conversation went like this:

Mark: Come on, baby, come on, we'll use protection. I won't tell anyone.

Jean: I just don't . . . I just can't.

Mark: Come on, you said you would.

Jean: I know I did, but I'm just . . . not ready. . . .

Seeing that Jean looked so uncomfortable, I stepped in and doubled with her:

Powell: I'm going to pretend I am another part of you and you correct me if I don't say what you feel. Okay?

Jean: Okay.

Powell: I feel very uncomfortable playing this role. Is that how I feel?

Jean: Yes.

Powell: I want to help myself, but . . .

Jean: A woman just can't come out and . . . I mean—it may sound crazy, but if a woman just says, "no way" people are going to think she's . . . she's . . . *a bitch . . . or a prude, or something.*

And there we have it. That statement epitomizes a fear American women have of asserting themselves about sexual issues. It is a terrible conflict for a heterosexual woman to think a man won't accept her if she shows strength. Yet strength is what any adult needs—to do a job successfully, to be a parent, and to remain steadfast through life's stresses. If you pretend to be weaker (or stronger) than you are, you attract people who will never really get along with you once you become yourself. When you behave in a healthy, confident way as an equal to others, you attract a different kind of person. As psychologist Abraham Maslow is reputed to have said of women, "Alleycats attract tomcats, and lionesses attract lions."

Mind Versus Body

Sex is one of the few areas in life in which you might really feel like doing something with your *body* that your *mind* knows is not good for you. Cravings for alcohol and unhealthy foods, as well as compulsive exercising, are probably the only drives that compare at all to a sexual situation. You want your passionate feelings to happen in the right time and place, but what do you need to *believe* in order to be convincing when you assert your sexual rights?

Family Scripts

Some therapists say that you are scripted in childhood for what you will do and say as an adult.[3] A life script is an early, unconscious program for what you will do with your life. As you grow, you learn how things happen, and after a while you quite naturally assume that's how things are *supposed* to happen. You have been given internal beliefs, a script that you tend to act out; you are on the stage of life, acting as you were taught to act, anticipating what you've been taught to expect. For example, you could probably write the rest of this scene from your own past experience:

You (as a little kid): Mom, where do babies come from?

Mom: I'll tell you later.

Or:

You: Dad, what's a condom?

Dad: You're too young to be talking about things like that (or fill in what your dad would have said).

If your parents were uncomfortable, you probably stopped asking. They might have been willing to hang in there anyway, but hearing their discomfort you still were *scripted*, "Don't talk about sex." You were also scripted either to stand up for yourself or to give in. An obedient child is a pleasure. Rebellion is annoying, if not infuriating, so most of us learned to squelch some of our own feelings in order to obey adults. We say you were scripted—to obey without question, or to reason with others who disagree; to please everyone whenever possible, or to be devious. Whether you are fifteen or fifty, you remember the scripts of your childhood.

Anya, for example, always tries to manipulate men by playing games with them. She believes in playing hard to get, but she also makes them think she likes them and enjoys pulling the rug out from under them periodically by dating someone else. Her mother manipulated her father all through Anya's childhood, and Anya watched and learned. Her mother even went so far as to advise her, "Never let a man know what you're thinking—keep the upper hand." Thus Anya was scripted to manipulate men.

Don watched his dad and uncles drink. He heard his mother and aunts complain about it but saw that they did nothing. He was scripted to "Stay drunk and be out of control," and he lived up to it when he reached his twenties. This way of life affected his lovemaking and also gave him an excuse to impose sex on his dates.

We were also scripted about pleasure. Some of us got the message "Have fun!" and some of us got the message "Fun is risky." Even if they were unsaid, very clear messages in our families taught us what to expect of sex when we became adults. A parent tries to hold back a child's interest in sexual activity by minimizing any talk about sexual pleasure. This is an effort to protect. But sometimes parents go overboard with warnings. No parent, even with the best intentions, can be certain of giving his child a positive script about sex. At first a child needs protection, but when he grows up he will need to view sex as a pleasure. So he may receive a confusing message: "Enjoy sex, but don't." Some other sexual messages are:

You'll turn out to be a whore just like your aunt.

I hope you'll sow your wild oats as I always wanted to.

Your body is important—take care of it and enjoy it.

No one needs to have said the words to you directly—you got the message. And the message may have stayed with you the rest of your life. Up until now.

Beliefs You Will Need

When your belief conflicts with what you are supposed to do, what you believe often wins. For example, if you really believe it's okay to make a mistake you can probably speak with ease in front of a group. But if you believe mistakes are terrible, you probably will not volunteer for any talking that would open you up to criticism.

If you are assertive you just naturally have a set of healthy beliefs. In a sense, you actually tell yourself healthy things—you have a running dialogue with yourself. For example, someone gets in front of you as you are waiting in line. "He's not supposed to do that, it isn't fair!" says a part of you. And this inner voice may spur you to take action.

Or you're preparing for a date with a new person and you're scared you will get sexual too quickly, as you have in the past. "Hope I can be careful," you say to yourself. And on another level you're probably saying, "I can't wait to touch him." Your passionate feelings tell you to do one thing, and your higher brain, capable of looking at long-range consequences, tells you to do another.

Or you're a male scripted to score. A woman is an object to conquer. You may hear yourself thinking, "What could I do to get her to go all the way?"

Usually we aren't even aware of them, but certain situations bring these beliefs to the conscious level of our thoughts. For example, you may believe, "It's embarrassing to talk about sex to my partner." You don't realize you believe this until there you are with her, intending to speak up, feeling awkward and unable to reach even the hemming and hawing stage. You're telling yourself how *awful* it is to talk about sex to your partner or you're telling yourself you'll *hurt her feelings*, or you'll look like a *fool*, or any number of things; and that all of those things are *mortifying*. Someone else, on the other hand, might believe it's okay to speak up, and have none of these painful emotions.

Albert Ellis, a psychologist who doesn't mince words, attacks clients' unhealthy beliefs, in psychotherapy.[4] He says that before we can stop ourselves from feeling painful emotions, we have to stop negative thoughts, because they *create* our negative emotions.

For example, let's say LaMar is getting ready for a date. He's been intending to discuss safer sex practices with this woman for a few days, since desire has reached the risky stage. His thought processes go something like this:

LaMar (Looking in the mirror, shaving.): God, I better tell her. (He pictures or hears himself beginning to talk about safer sex or hears his voice saying it.) She'll think I'm a wimp. I should (he imagines her face looking disapproving), but I can't. I can't stand to think about it. She doesn't have any diseases. (He turns on the radio.)

What LaMar is saying to himself is, "It's terrible and awful if I talk to my date about sexual protection. If I do, I'll be embarrassed and feel dumb, and men are supposed to be in control. She may be uncomfortable and the whole thing will be a terrible catastrophe." Telling himself these things causes LaMar's heart to beat a little faster and his muscles to tense. He actually flinches a little as he shaves. A cognitive therapist in the Ellis tradition would probably train LaMar to catch himself in these negative beliefs and self-talk. Catastrophizing happens when we tell ourselves the worst thing is going to happen, such as: It would be terrible and a catastrophe if:

I can't think of the right words to say.
I made a mistake.
Somebody got mad at me.
This relationship ended.
Somebody criticized me.
I showed my emotions.

Such a therapist would train LaMar to substitute a more rational thought, something like this: "It might be somewhat awkward to talk to a woman about sex at this stage. If she doesn't like what I say, I might feel uneasy for a short time. However, she might respond positively and appreciate my courage in speaking up. If she does not, I can survive a little discomfort in order to help us be sexually safe."

Sexually assertive people believe in the sexual rights in Chapter 2. They might differ here or there on these rights, but they are generally clear. When they are in a sexual situation, they might not be thinking consciously about their rights, but they're aware of them at all times. This may not be true of you. You may be confused easily when another person provokes guilt in you or threatens you. But if you're clear on your sexual rights, you believe the following:

1. I never have to please another person sexually unless the idea truly appeals to me.

2. If anyone rejects me for my sexual beliefs or preferences, I can survive and very likely find another person.

3. I am not a child who needs an adult to help me survive; I am an adult and I can take care of myself even if I have to be alone for a while.

4. I am capable of speaking up when I see a sexual risk, or a chance to improve my sexual relationship.

If, deep down, you believe those things, you will feel calmer and more able to cope.

To further prepare yourself to be assertive, you might repeat to yourself some of the affirmations that Pamela Butler, Ph.D., advises in her book about assertion :

It isn't awful to make a mistake.
I'm not going to apologize for where I am now.
It's okay to feel nervous. That's part of entering a new territory.
There is no perfect way of saying this.
If my mind has gone blank, it's okay to say "My mind has gone blank."

Common Beliefs about Sex

How healthy are your sexual beliefs? You need all the insight you can get about your sexual attitudes. Mark the following True or False:

___ I can't control my sex drive.

___ Chastity is bad for me and I can't stand it.

___ Truly liberated men (women) have sex whenever they want.

___ A virgin has not really entered adulthood.

___ Having sex is the only way to hang on to a prospective mate.

___ If I refuse sex I'll lose the other person, and that's disastrous.

___ If the other person gets mad at me when I refuse sex or ask for protection, it's awful and horrible.

___ If my partner doesn't like something I say or do, it's a calamity and I feel awful.

___ If I am rejected because of my beliefs I'll never find another person to care about.

___ If my partner puts me down because I refuse sex, it's a horrible humiliation that would not happen to a real man.

___ If I stop when I'm very aroused, I can't stand it.

___ Discussing safer sex is unromantic and/or naughty.

___ It's unfeminine to insist on something with a man you care about; he'll love you less if you do.

___ Everybody else has a great sex life but me.

___ I can't exist without someone to love.

___ I need sex to prove I am attractive.

___ I need sex to prove I'm a real man.

___ Sex is my most important need.

___ Mature adults have sex as soon as they feel attraction.

What was your score? All of the above beliefs are unhealthy. They aren't the truth. They are just opinions that some people have. Learn to rephrase your negative statements. For example, let's say you tell yourself, "It's terrible and awful if my partner puts me down when I bring up the subject of sexually transmitted disease." A healthier statement would be, "It would be very nice (pleasant, comfortable) if my partner responded the way I want. However, since life is not perfect, he may possibly try to persuade me to his way of thinking instead. While I might feel uncomfortable for a while, I can certainly stand it in order to keep myself healthy."

Try to evaluate your sexual beliefs. Go back to Chapter 2 and read the sexual rights again. Do you believe you have the sexual rights discussed?

Beliefs about Your Health

Experts have studied people to find out what beliefs cause them to take the best care of their health. Those who are most careful about preventing AIDS tend to believe the following:[6]

1. I am susceptible to AIDS.
2. AIDS is a severe disease.
3. AIDS is preventable.
4. I should take active care of my health.

People who don't believe all of these statements obviously aren't going to try as hard to prevent AIDS.

Self-Esteem

"You got me all worked up, and you say *NO?*" says one man in my class role-plays. His partner, a woman, is looking at him uncomfortably and is momentarily speechless. At this point I often go up to the speechless partner and point to the top of her head. "What happens next," I say, "depends entirely on what's going on in here."

That's right. Because if her self-concept and self-esteem are low, she is at risk. If you don't think you deserve something, you won't assert yourself to get it.

What is self-esteem? The phrase refers simply to how much you value yourself, and it goes along with trusting yourself, not exploiting anyone, and caring about other people. It's terribly unfair, but low self-esteem is correlated with a huge number of life problems, including being prejudiced and failing to help others in emergencies. It is also involved in all kinds of sexual difficulties, such as exhibitionism and obscene phone calling. People with low self-esteem may treat themselves with disrespect and often see themselves as unable to resist persuasion.

Your first responsibility in this world is to take care of yourself. If you don't think you are worth it, you won't do a good job of it. The easiest way to feel you're worth taking care of is to have been raised by wonderful parents who loved you and set limits. They would have had no significant problems with self-esteem themselves. If you had no major childhood illnesses, learning disabilities, abuse, or other traumas, that helps your self-esteem as well. (Parents aren't responsible for everything.) Since these ideal parents and trauma-free childhoods have been denied to most of us, we have the job of improving our self-esteem on our own.

Sometimes life events just challenge us and we rise to the occasion. We cope with problems, and our self-esteem improves. We accomplish things or help someone, and our confidence rises. But sometimes we need professional help to get over the damage of the past. Consult the Appendix for sources of help to improve your self-esteem.

How to Reward Yourself

One of psychology's greatest wisdoms is that behavior that is rewarded tends to happen more often. You can apply that rather obvious truth to mental rewards. You can reward yourself. Here is how this might work:

Steve has had some near misses with sexually transmitted diseases. In college, he contracted gonorrhea, and it was slow in responding to treatment, but he finally tested out okay. He once got his girlfriend pregnant in high school and she had an abortion. He s begun to realize that he needs to deal with his sexuality differently. He's just begun dating Vicki, a very sexy-looking woman whom he finds terrifically attractive. She's making every attempt to get him to have intercourse, although it's only their third date. However, he knows nothing about her sexual past or her sexual opinions. He gets clues that she has had lots of other sexual partners. He's finding this really frustrating, and he's afraid she will shame him or he will feel stupid if he turns her down. He knows condoms aren't risk-free and isn't even ready for a condom mentally, but physically he's ready for intercourse.

So, maybe even shaking with passion, he says, "Hey, Vicki, you really turn me on. But I want to slow this down a little. I feel like we're on a roller-coaster here." Vicki replies, touching him suggestively, "Good! Let's take a ride!" Steve gets up and pulls her up from the couch by the hands. He takes a deep breath. "Vicki, I—I want to take my time here, for you and me both. Why don't we go to a movie or something?" Vicki searches his face. She seems to see his determination. "Okay," she says.

That night when Steve gets home he still remembers how much he wanted Vicki, but he knows he avoided his previous problems. If he ever catches himself thinking how embarrassing it was, he quickly corrects himself: That was rough, but I did the smart thing.

Steve is using the disease-prevention technique of self-reward. Even if she had reacted by putting him down, he could still tell himself he did the right thing. Whenever you do something that is good for you, take the time to congratulate yourself. It raises your self-esteem. Your culture is not going to reward you for being sexually assertive, and if you are a young male, your friends probably won't either. Right after you do something sexually assertive, you could say something to yourself to remind and reinforce yourself:

"Wow! That was tough, but I did refuse to take a risk, even if he (she) wasn't happy."

"That was great; tonight I explained my opinions about getting sexually involved on a casual date."

"It's been three months since I did anything risky."

Or just plain, "Good for me!"

It's often even better if you can reward yourself out loud, letting the other person know:

A: I'm glad I told you how I feel. That was hard to do.

B: I'm glad, too.

A: I'm getting better at it.

Even if the other person doesn't agree with your decision, you can reward yourself for being sexually assertive:

A: I'm glad I told you how I feel.

B: Well, it sure ruined my evening.

A: I'm sorry you don't like what I said. But I've tried so hard to get the nerve to speak up. I really needed to tell you that because it's been worrying me.

We're very critical of conceited people. We don't like anyone to be too uppity around us; we feel inadequate, perhaps. Yet, ironically, most of us spend our lives trying to gain more self-confidence. That puts us in a bind—we can't be humble and very confident at the same time. I think there's no real danger that people who gain confidence will become obnoxiously conceited. So, compliment yourself in any way you can when you're being assertive, and even ask some significant other person to help:

A: Honey, you know I've been trying hard to tell you that I want to keep using protection every time we make love.

B: Yeah, I know.

A: When I mention the subject, you always look so serious. Would you try to give me a little encouragement?

B: Sure, I'll try.

Real Courage

Thousands of moments in a little boy's life tell him what a man should be. The self-esteem of American males gets tied up quite early with power, conquest, and bravery. But men especially need to reconsider their definition of bravery. When a man speaks up to defend himself from sexual problems, he needs to congratulate himself. It is brave to speak up against things that hurt you or your society. I know some wonderful men with the courage to speak out about important issues regardless of who agrees with them. It doesn't take courage just to copy some muscle-bound macho hero saying yes to every female who offers her body. The mass media show no models of honest, realistic sexual behavior for young males to imitate. Didn't James Bond have sex without a second thought with scores of gorgeous women? Didn't just about every TV or film hero you've ever seen take every sexy woman up on her offer in less time than it takes to shake hands?

I've seen male students in their thirties who feel secure and experienced enough to role-play very assertively and frankly about sex. But how should the frustrated teenage boy feel who takes a deep breath and tells a girl he needs to get to know her better? Far from feeling unmanly, he should compliment himself: "I'm strong. What a man!"

As for women, they are often afraid to take a sexual stand that could in any way be described as courageous. Succeeding chapters will explain skills to overcome this fear.

Guided Imagery

Fantasizing can serve not only as a substitute for something sexual you want to do, it can also be a rehearsal for what you are *planning* to do. That is, you're more likely to do something if you have imagined it beforehand; the images are a first step toward the reality. Professionals advise that people rehearse mentally before engaging in any important new actions. Psychotherapists often help clients to learn a new behavior by helping them to imagine themselves doing it. Athletic trainers may help athletes mentally rehearse a game or a race. A speech teacher may ask students to see and listen to themselves giving the important presentation. This is called *visualization* or *guided imagery*. You can use your sexual thoughts and fantasies to help yourself in the same way. Sex educators recommend that you practice healthy scripts rather than fantasizing unhealthy or risky scenes.

It's fun for most people to have sexual fantasies before a date or sexual encounter, and it might help you to observe how you fantasize. You need only a few moments to include safer sex practices in your fantasies. There is research to show that people who substitute safer-sex fantasies have a lower rate of sexually transmitted disease than people who continue daydreaming about risky sex.[7] For example, if you think it's best for you to just kiss and keep your clothes on when you have a particular date, imagine yourself doing that. Imagine when the other person shows an interest in doing more; picture, or hear yourself saying and doing what you need to do at that point. Wild fantasies are fine if you're able to do what you want when it comes down to real life, but if you're having any trouble with self-control, fantasizing risky activities is risky in itself. It's like a mental rehearsal. If you are involved in a relationship other than a monogamous one with someone you know for sure is uninfected, fantasize about using condoms correctly before you make love. It's not Hollywood, but it's still sexy.

Thought-Stopping

Most of us have been bothered by some of our thoughts at times. Maybe they weren't even sexual. Maybe you made a mistake and later said to yourself, "How stupid, how stupid!" You wanted to stop calling yourself stupid, but the thought kept popping into your mind. Or maybe you went over and over the mistake in your thoughts and felt the embarrassment or humiliation all over again.

Psychologists have come up with some clever and simple ways to change your thoughts. Hang on, because this is going to sound far-fetched. But evidence indicates that people can decrease and sometimes completely eliminate negative thoughts by yelling at themselves.

Yes, it is true. These are ways you can punish away an undesired thought. It's done like this: Every time you have a negative thought, you yell, "Stop!" In this way, you punish yourself for having a dysfunctional thought. Yell out loud if you're alone or yell inside your head if you're with others. (Even your dog may not appreciate a sudden shock.) That means you yell *every time* you catch yourself having the undesirable thought. It's best to immediately replace that thought with a positive one, opposite to the bad thought. At first it may seem that this simple technique does not work, but if you use it faithfully it should begin to take hold.

Take Lavonne, for example, who has been trying to get up the nerve to discuss condoms with her partner. Whenever Lavonne even thinks about the condom conversation, she says to herself, "He's going to get so mad!" Rationally, she knows that she must protect herself by discussing condoms. So every time she catches herself thinking of his anger, she yells, "No!" to herself. Gradually the thought diminishes.

Every time you banish the undesirable thought, you should make yourself substitute a healthy one. After Lavonne yells, "No!" inside her head, she immediately says, "I'm helping us both. I'm doing him a favor, too." When she imagines sex with him, she imagines it only with a condom. This makes it easier to talk to her partner about using one.

Either that or snap a rubber band. Yes, if you prefer another of these punishment techniques, instead of yelling you may put a rubber band on your wrist and snap it hard every time you think an undesirable thought. I'm not worried that this technique will sweep the country, but it's actually proved quite an effective aid for treating certain habits.

The Parts of You

There is another insight that can help some people to feel more secure. To learn this you'll need a little background. We all have various "parts" in our personalities. This does not mean we have multiple personalities like the famous Sybil or Eve. Because normally, unlike Eve, we know about the different parts. For example, on many Friday afternoons part of you says, "Finish your work," and another part says, "Let's get out of here and enjoy." If you're kissing someone passionately, one part is probably screaming, "Where is the nearest private place where we can do whatever we want?" And another part (even if it seems like a weak little voice), may be saying, "I should . . . " (fill in the blank with the rational statements that are almost drowned out by the other part of you).

The various voices in us develop in childhood. Millions of people have grown up feeling both unloved and unsafe due to physically or emotionally scary things that happened to them. For example, Jerry grew up with a passive father and a controlling, seductive mother. Although she did not actually touch Jerry in a seductive way, during his adolescence she often invited him in to talk to her as she put on her makeup, naked from the waist up. She told him lovingly that, when he was born, his aunts looked at him nude and said he would make some woman very happy someday. She mentioned wistfully times when he was nude as a child. She told him his father was sexually inadequate. She was jealous of his girlfriends.

During this time, his father was cold and hostile to Jerry. He had nowhere to turn. His father hated him, and his mother cared in a controlling, seductive way. His childhood was painful and lonely. He struggled with the confusing ideas about sex and love that he learned growing up. As an adult, he suffered from the most acute feelings of loneliness and pain, but he also was seductive with girls around the age of puberty.

When scary or hurtful things happen to a little child, these events can cause the person to become partly stuck in childhood. That is, feelings of fear, anger, or hurt felt in childhood keep coming up in adulthood *with the same intensity that the helpless child felt back then.* Even though it's not appropriate for an adult to feel so scared, helpless, or abandoned, she still has all the child's strong and painful feelings. The transactional analysts believe we are always operating in either our Adult, Child, or Parent state. We might say, in the words of TA, that the individual is "operating in her child" at such times. She is bypassing the more adult and nurturant parts of herself because they weren't there when she was little.

You can see how the child part took over in the life of Luis, who was compulsively sexual. He engaged in sex at virtually every opportunity. He knew it was risky, and he even knew some friends who had been infected with HIV. But he desperately wanted to be loved. He grew up with very critical, rejecting parents. His father was an alcoholic who beat him. Whenever he got into a sexual situation that could involve risk, he felt helpless and little, as if he had to do whatever his partner wanted so he wouldn't relive those old feelings. After years of sexual troubles, he decided to take responsibility for those things and consult a professional for help.

After Luis went into therapy, he began to understand his sexual compulsions. Whenever he was out with someone, just at the critical moment of deciding to go further sexually, he began to be aware of scary, awful feelings. He felt that he *had* to go ahead and have sex, regardless of safety or any other consideration. What he learned in therapy was, "I'm not little. I'm not stuck with two unloving parents anymore. I have a grownup part of myself now that can take care of me and help me find love and avoid pain. That caring part of me is right there when I'm making sexual decisions, if I can just listen to it."

We all have a little child element incorporated in our personalities. For the lucky few, that aspect grew up so secure that as adults they never get those helpless childhood feelings of rage, desertion, shame, or terror. But for most of us, stressful experiences trigger the little kid's old, painful feelings. On the other hand, we all have a grownup part that we lacked in childhood. We all are more capable of protecting ourselves than that helpless child was, but sometimes we don't realize it. When adults are unaware of their own adult power it can cause them to feel:

- totally alone with the feelings of an abandoned child rather than the temporary loneliness of an adult.
- as scared as if they might die, when they are really adult enough to stay safe.
- angry enough to kill someone, and afraid they have no control over their anger.

- terrified when someone else is angry at them, as if they were to be killed, rather than only a bit anxious as a secure adult might be.

Past feelings influence your sex life. These strong feelings can encourage hasty sexual decisions. If you are not keeping yourself safe sexually, if you repeatedly take sexual risks or cause yourself other sexual problems, you may want to check out your thoughts and feelings. Could it be that just when you're on the verge of deciding to go further sexually, you have the strong emotions you had as a child?

- I'm scared to back out now or he'll be mad and that's awful and terrible.
- At last someone loves me—I'll do whatever he says.
- If I just please her, I'll finally be loved.

Learning to get past your childhood fears can be an important step toward protecting yourself sexually. If you think your fears are causing you to make unwise decisions, you may want to find some professional help (see Appendix).

Feeling Down

Sometimes your mood puts you at risk for making stupid sexual decisions. When you are depressed, be extra protective of yourself, because you may be more vulnerable to sexual mistakes at such times. Normal adults have a part of their personalities that can watch out for them when they're depressed. Adults don't need a parent to take care of them anymore, but they do need to develop a "parent" within themselves. When you're lonely or depressed, you need to be wary of the little tricks your mind can play on you. Because at such times the childlike irrationality in you may want sex for reassurance, regardless of your age.

You could talk to yourself when you catch yourself really down and say, "Self, I need to watch it here; I feel really defenseless. If someone should get sexually involved with me right now, I might be putty in her hands. I need to take special care of myself right now." It's as if you were carrying something very delicate down the stairs. You might have bounded up and down the stairs when your hands were empty. But when you're carrying a valuable china dish, you watch your step, and remind yourself that you're carrying precious cargo. When you're feeling depressed, look out for yourself. You are precious cargo.

Donna's experience shows how mood and self-esteem affect sexual decisions. She had never been close to a man. Her father left when she was nine and doesn't contact her. Donna is flirtatious and enjoys dressing up, going out, and meeting men. For a while she dated a new man every couple of weeks and almost always had intercourse with him. After about four years of this behavior, she began to be alarmed about the kind of men with whom she was sleeping. She admitted to her friends that sex was like a hug to her—she didn't need sex as much as human touch.

"I felt so alone in this world," she said. "I couldn't tell the difference between sex and love. It was a warm body to be close to." Donna realized that not only was sex not helping, in this case it was putting her at risk for other serious consequences. Getting sex is not the same as getting love. Next time you think you want sex, take a deep breath and pause for a moment. Ask yourself, "If someone held me and hugged me, would I feel mostly satisfied? What else could I do to take care of myself right now?" Try to make sure of what you want before you decide that sex is what you need.

Self-Hypnosis

There are entertainers (stage hypnotists), and there are competent, well-trained professionals who use clinical hypnosis. Some of their clinical methods guide people in behavior changes, such as control of overeating and smoking. Put simply, hypnosis can change your behaviors and thoughts by getting through on a very deep level of which you are usually unaware.

It is possible to help strengthen yourself with some of the self-hypnotic techniques used by clinical hypnosis. You need not go into an actual trance to borrow a few of their techniques. So as to concentrate fully, you should close your eyes and use these methods when you're not driving or doing anything else that requires your attention.

For example, Spiegel and Spiegel are psychiatrists who have helped numerous people quit smoking. They designed a kind of self-statement for smokers that can be helpful in changing sexual behavior. For smokers, it went like this:

> *Smoking is a poison to my body.*
> *I need my body to live.*
> *I owe my body respect and protection.*[8]

To use this technique to with sexual behavior, you have to rephrase it to fit your situation. Suppose, for example, that Rick engages in casual sex whenever he feels like it. Maybe he's an attractive person who can find numerous partners. He's worried because he has had curable STDs and knows he could become infected with the incurable ones. He needs a reminder, to program his unconscious a bit by keeping healthy, self-protective thoughts foremost in his mind. So when he wakes up in the morning, and goes to sleep at night, and before he enters any situation that might tempt him to take risks, he closes his eyes, breathes slowly, and repeats to himself,

"Casual sex is a risk to my body."

"I need my body to live."

"I owe my body respect and protection."

Nina phrases her reminder a different way. Earlier in her life she had a sexual relationship she regrets. She intends to remain abstinent until she is in a very serious relationship. She wants to marry and have children. She knows that even curable STDs might leave her sterile. She is a passionate person and enjoys non-penetrative sexual activities. She repeats an affirmation to herself sometimes before she goes out on a date:

"Sex without love is a danger to my body and my feelings."

"I need my body to live and have children."

"I owe my whole body respect and protection."

This statement of her rational knowledge supports her and protects her from physical impulses. She stops, closes her eyes for a moment, and repeats her reminder to herself before she goes out with her date.

Although this may sound far out to some readers, affirmations are accepted in the field of mental health as one way to shut out dysfunctional thoughts and concentrate. To some, it might be like a prayer. To others, it's like repeating a poem. Some people enjoy developing the inner self. People who compulsively take sexual risks may especially need frequent reminders of their inner strengths, just as an alcoholic may need to attend frequent AA meetings to keep sobriety foremost in her mind.

The Holistic Approach

Research shows that frequent reminders have helped a number of people to avoid STDs. Rather than try to help ourselves with just one technique or one viewpoint, it is better to bring in a variety of props and aids to healthy behavior. This is called the *holistic approach*. You can pick and choose from a number of ways to help yourself. One person may put reminders on the mirror or refrigerator:

I Have Untapped Strength

Will I Feel Good the Next Morning?

You can attach little reminders here and there if you find them helpful. Even a symbol, such as a picture of yourself at a happy time, can be your private reminder. Some people arrange for healthy reminders by joining groups that help them get past disturbing sexual messages. There are support groups, for example, for sexual addicts, incest survivors, and rape survivors. (See Appendix for ways to find those groups.) We are tribal animals, and the lack of a caring group is one of the most profound losses in industrialized societies. We need support from others, whether it's family, church, temple, or friends. Perhaps someday there will be groups where anyone needing support can talk about sexual concerns.

Whatever you choose to do, be aware that *your mind is already programmed sexually*. Your childhood has given you various sexual messages, and you have kept many of them throughout your teenage or adult life. Now you may want to add to those messages or try to change some of them to help yourself and to make the sexual decisions you have rationally decided are best for you.

Which Were You Scripted to Believe?

Somewhere in your life you picked up messages about sex and yourself as a sexual being. Check those ideas that were in your script, regardless of whether parents or others intended you to get that message. The script is a message in their words, even if they did not say it openly. To help you get the idea of a script, imagine that as you grew up, you were in the theater of life, and deep down the directors really wanted you to act as if:

___ 1. Sex is a joyous gift.

___ 2. Sex is dangerous.

___ 3. Sex is shameful.

___ 4. Sex is somewhat embarrassing.

___ 5. Sex is okay between married people.

___ 6. Sex is dirty.

___ 7. Sex is not to be discussed in my presence.

___ 8. You can do anything sexual you want, and we'll look the other way.

___ 9. You'd better behave yourself sexually, or else.

___10. You'd better stay out of trouble and don't tell me anything I don't want to hear.

___11. Sex is an important thing, and you should enjoy it in safe circumstances.

___12. I know you'll conduct yourself properly.

___13. I get a vicarious thrill hearing about your sex life.

___14. Don't use sex the way I have.

___15. Sex is something you'll learn about later.

___16. I'll wink and look the other way if you have some fun.

___17. Sex is just a normal part of life.

___18. Sex is a sacred gift from God, to be shared with one person.

___19. Sex is confusing.

___20. The only way to show love and affection is to be sexual.

___21. Having sex is the same thing as being used.

Notes

1. David Burns, *Feeling Good: The New Mood Therapy* (New York: New American Library, 1980), 234.

2. Joseph H. Pleck, Freya L. Sonenstein, and Leighton C. Ku, "Masculinity Ideology: Its Impact on Adolescent Males' Heterosexual Relationships," *Journal of Social Issues* 49, no. 3 (1993): 11–29.

3. Barbara Engler, *Personality Theories: An Introduction.* (Boston: Houghton Mifflin Co., 1995), 251.

4. Engler, *Personality Theories: An Introduction* 423.

5. Pamela Butler, *Self-Assertion for Women* (San Francisco: HarperSanFrancisco, 1992), 50–51.

6. Robert Allard, "Beliefs about AIDS as Determinants of Preventive Practices and of Support for Coercive Measures," *American Journal of Public Health* 79, no. 4 (April 1989): 448.

7. Jeffrey A. Kelly and Janet S. St. Lawrence, *Behavioral Group Intervention to Teach AIDS Risk Reduction Skills* (Jackson, Miss.: University of Mississippi Medical School, 1990), 43.

8. David Spiegel and Herbert Spiegel, *Trance and Treatment: Clinical Uses of Hypnosis* (New York: Basic Books, 1978), 215.

Part II

How to Respond to Persuasion

4

Standing Up To Verbal Pressure

. . . a time to embrace,
and a time to refrain from embracing.
—ECCLESIASTES 3:5

Do all cultures have sexual pressure? Some wise scholar has pointed out that we can't really know about people's sexual activities in other societies. These faraway folks may not hanker to tell some visiting anthropologist what they do in private. But as far as we know, men have historically taken the role of the sexual pursuer. Today women are encouraged to pursue men as well. Just about anyone could find himself being sexually pressured. Most societies do not promote getting sex by trickery or manipulation as much as we do in our media. "Wooing" someone with flowers, gifts, or compliments has been replaced in the media by the slick line. And the polite suitor has given way to the smooth operator.

The Customs of Sexual Pressure

From the sixties through the eighties, the pill, abortion, and other technological changes gave people the impression that they could have sex without paying a high price. At the same time, we lost our strong standards or customs to fall back on as excuses to refuse sex. Although pregnancies did occur, the following was a common scenario in the fifties for a high school or college couple who had dated just a few times:

He: (Puts his hand on her breast.)

53

She: (Likes it, but feels worried about her reputation, the prospect of intercourse, the possibility of pregnancy, her marketability as a marriage mate if she is promiscuous, his opinion of her.)

She: (Moving his hand away), No, I—I can't.

He: Why not?

She: I just can't, that's all.

He: (Tries again more tentatively.)

She: Stop it!

He: I'm sorry.

Many couples repeated this scenario, and perhaps progressed sexually, depending on how she felt about him. The use of force on a date, while it did happen, was not as common as it is today. He knew what her standards were likely to be; all "nice girls" supposedly had those standards.

These were certainly not the "good old days", but sexual standards were not often questioned in public. The ideas that nice girls don't or sex should wait until marriage have now been openly questioned throughout our society. A woman on a date can't usually claim some strong belief in virginity based on the values of her community. She has to fend for herself and come up with her own reasons. More experienced women can rely on even fewer excuses. Many of the reasons women once used are no longer valid. "It will ruin my reputation" is hardly a major concern in a society where sexual intercourse is taken for granted among most singles. Although it was once considered the woman's responsibility to set sexual limits, now no one is quite certain whose role it is. Standards for men have not changed that much, and statistics show it. The greatest increase in premarital sex is among women. Most young men are still influenced by the standard that they should be out trying to score, and now it has become an open competition about which many young men brag to each other. Because young males place such a high premium on sexual conquests, it is often very difficult for them to turn down a sexual opportunity while still maintaining their composure and self-assurance. Men are supposed to:

- pressure for sex when they can; and
- appear ready to accept just about any sexual offer.

This pressure to be a stud and prove one's masculinity changes the way sexual pressure occurs in our country. Listen to the words of one male college student describing what goes on between a man and a woman:

*A man is supposed to view a date with a woman as a premeditated scheme
for getting the most sex out of her. Everything he does, he judges in terms*

of one criterion— "getting laid." He's supposed to constantly pressure her to see how far he can get. She is his adversary, his opponent in a battle, and he begins to view her as a prize, an object, not a person. While she's dreaming about love, he's thinking about how to conquer her.

Sexual pressure has become big business. Not just courting, but pushing, insisting, even getting rough. You see it in ads, in films and TV, and in songs. The lyrics of some of today's songs actually describe, in detail, how much fun it is to rape a woman. In order to resist sexual pressure, singles of any age need to learn how to recognize manipulation and sexual deception. They also need to learn how to give clear yes or no messages to a potential sex partner. In this chapter we'll talk about what you could say when someone tries to persuade you with words to go further than you want to go. But this does not involve resisting physical force. It concerns only what you say to resist being verbally pressured into sex.

Using Your Higher Brain Power

Let us not underestimate the higher brain's ability to overpower the sex drive. Although nature's concern is with the human species, your own survival has a higher priority to you than survival of the human race. If the bear came over the mountain while your ancestors were becoming sexually aroused, their sexual responses stopped and they got out of there. Because of this safety feature, you have inherited the capacity to postpone or refuse sex. The turnoff mechanism was an advantage to survival.

In some societies, people still use great sexual restraint. Prior to the use of the birth control pill, American females more commonly tried to postpone sex until marriage, and many succeeded. Of those who did not postpone, millions had fewer partners before marriage than unmarried people today, and fewer diseases.

Brainwashing

We've learned to think of sex as a process of being overwhelmed by intense passion without first thinking ahead. And we do have a capacity for the most delightful and delicious passionate feelings with no rational thought involved. It's wonderful to feel swept away, at least at that moment. But a kind of unintentional brainwashing also occurs in our society that few of us criticize, in the hundreds of portrayals of people being carried away by passion. Sex is the only appetite that we encourage one another to unleash. We don't accept dramas about ravenously hungry people who grab food and eat with no preliminaries. Some kind of preparatory behavior precedes eating, such as picking up a knife and fork, or asking someone to pass the food. But even in novels, the characters go straight to intercourse with no preliminaries. They never ask for a condom; unrestrained passion is the rule.

The fantasy of wildly abandoned sexual freedom is used in ads about cars and clothes, and it sells films, books, and movies. How do you protect yourself from sexual problems in the face of this distorted viewpoint?

Recognizing Pressure Lines

In the past few years I've polled my students about the best sexual pressure lines they've ever heard. I explain that a line is manipulative and dishonest, spoken by a person who is trying to get sex by devious means, whereas if someone says the same thing sincerely it is not manipulation. Younger and inexperienced people are usually the most prone to fall for these lines, but in the heat of passion or infatuation, even people in middle age can be vulnerable. For example, *I love you* could be the best words you've ever heard, and part of a beautiful relationship. But if you're out with someone who has been through everyone in your group sexually, who's never shown any interest in you as a person, and who, necking passionately with you, says, "I love you," doubt it.

Obviously the context in which someone makes a loving remark will provide clues about whether it's true. But being "in lust" or "in love" leaves you open to believing statements that look humorous on the printed page. Over the years, my surveys have come up with a long list of lines, most of which fall into definite patterns:

Line That Declares Love and Caring
"I don't want to have sex with you—I want to make love to you."

Lines That Reassure You about the Negative Consequences
"Don't worry, I'm sterile."

"You can't get pregnant the first time." (This is not true.)

"Don't worry—I'll pull out." (Withdrawal before ejaculation will not prevent pregnancy, because some semen can leak out earlier.)

"I won't tell anyone."

"I'll respect you even more."

Line That Threatens You with Rejection
"If you don't have sex, I'll find someone who will."

Lines That Attempt to Gain Sympathy
("Start crying if she says no—it works," says one student.)

"Now you have me hot and bothered."

"I'm a virgin and I've got six months to live."

"If a man gets too frustrated, it can fall off."

Line That Flatters
"You're one of the most beautiful women I've ever seen and I would be honored to spend the night with you."

Lines That Attempt to Put Down the Refuser
"You're such a bitch."

"You obviously have no respect for your body."

"Grow up, Pollyanna."

"Are you frigid?"

"You're really old-fashioned."

"You're not normal."

"Are you gay?"

"You're a virgin? Get serious!"

Lines That Stress the Beautiful Experience Being Missed
"Our relationship will grow stronger."

"Life is so short—let's make the most of it."

"Our relationship really needs to move on."

Lines That Might Settle for Less
"Won't you just lie there?"

"I don't want to do anything. I just want to lie next to you."

Lines That Attempt to be Logical But Aren't
"We're both married, so what's the problem?"

"Don't worry, I'm a doctor."

"If you don't like it, we won't have to do it again."

"You're my girlfriend—it's your obligation."

Line That Attempts to Answer the Religious Argument
"If God knew how good it was going to be, he'd let you."

Line that Suggests a Business Arrangement
"I'll let your drug debt slide if you sleep with me."

Lines That Are Totally Transparent ·
(If you believe either of these, you are extremely vulnerable to deception and might need to seek counseling to avoid being exploited.)

"I'll say I love you after we do it."

"I swear I'll get a divorce."

The World's Most Common Line
"If you loved me, you would."

Many of these lines are hilarious when taken out of a passionate sexual context. It's hard to believe that anyone would fall for them. But in the midst of passion, some of them seem, if not perfectly appropriate, at least temporarily believable.

Sol Gordon is a sex educator who combines academic knowledge with a down-to-earth approach in his book, *Seduction Lines Heard 'Round the World and Answers You Can Give.* He's quick on the uptake and recommends humorous retorts for various situations, mostly for people who are interested in turning off someone else's advances:

> *Female: "Sex isn't such a big deal. What are you waiting for?"*
> *Male: "I'm waiting for someone it's a big deal with."*
>
> *Female: "You should be flattered. I don't give my body to everyone."*
> *Male: "I wouldn't want to ruin your record."*
>
> *Male: "I feel like an animal when I'm around you."*
> *Female: "Should I spread some newspaper?"*[1]

Not everyone can think as fast as Sol Gordon or be that witty. It may not be a problem to use put-down retorts if the person is someone to whom you are not attracted, but when you are attracted (and maybe aroused), that person's lines may have more effect on you. You may tend to believe the lines because

- you are so aroused you'd love an excuse to proceed.
- you are so crazy about her you'd believe anything she said.
- you have come from a caring family background where people told the truth, and you just naturally believe it when someone says something loving to you.

Remember, recent surveys show that up to one-half of young Americans *admit* they will lie to get sex. (That's who actually admit it—we believe that the number who really *would* lie is much larger.) In one study, 68 percent of men and 59 percent of women college students said they had been sexually involved with more than one person and their partner did not know.[2] No doubt many singles in their thirties and forties would also mislead their partners. Even though men are the traditional seducers, women don't always tell the truth either. Some women have lied to entrap or hurt someone.

You may use what I'm saying to shore up cynical beliefs about why you should never trust anyone. If you think men or women are untrustworthy and relationships are always risky, you can quote parts of this book and reinforce that belief. But that is not the point. There is a wide range of people with whom you could form deep and loyal relationships. There are truthful people who wouldn't intentionally lie to hurt someone. But I'm trying to get you to become a bit skeptical if you're an overly trusting type. Learn to tell the difference between safe and unsafe sexual situations.

Ideal Sexual Assertion

In their manual *Behavioral Group Intervention to Teach AIDS Reduction Skills*, Jeffrey Kelly and Janet St. Lawrence list some important things you need to include if you're trying to be sexually assertive.[3] These techniques are based on learning theory, and they are scientifically sound ways to change behavior. They are not for situations where the partner is attempting to force you against your will. For other times, Kelly and St. Lawrence suggest that you:

1. *Acknowledge the other person's position*: That is, if you're in a situation where another person is pushing you with words, you can let him know you understand his viewpoint:

   "I know you'd like to keep going."
   "I know you don't like condoms."
   "I hear you, you think people should have sex whenever they want to, no matter how long they've known each other."

2. *Clearly refuse the other person's unreasonable demand*:

   "I won't have intercourse outside of a committed relationship."
   "I won't have sex without a condom."

3. *Explain the reason you are refusing the unreasonable request*:

   "Because I think it's too risky for disease."
   "Because I would not be comfortable with myself if I did."
   "Because it's against my religious beliefs."

Kelly and St. Lawrence further suggest that you tell your partner whether there's an alternative or solution acceptable to you. That is, if you won't do A or B to get sexual satisfaction, is there a safer alternative? If so, be specific when talking to your partner. And remember, a casual partner may disagree, but a person who is a good prospect for a relationship will not treat you with disrespect when you're asking for safer sex.

Your Policy Statement

If you were about to climb a mountain cliff with someone you did not know—where there was some danger, but reaching the top might be exhilarating—would you just tie on the ropes and take off up the cliff with her? No, you'd probably check out what kind of person she is, how she feels about climbing, who's going to go first, how much you might help each other. To begin with, you might tell her what you think about climbing cliffs. And you'd be looking quite carefully at her gear to see whether it was adequate for your protection as well as hers. You would listen carefully to her policy about safety.

Schools, churches, and even countries make policy statements. They spend much time perfecting these statements, and the good policy statements are as precise as possible. Long experience has taught them the importance of taking a clear stand on vital issues.

People who know they're close to becoming sexually involved need to let their partners know their policies about sex. Your date can no longer assume that you hold the policy "Nice women don't and men probably will." If you are older or divorced, you have no doubt realized that many dates assume you are sexually available. Women now have another kind of equality with men; now neither one has a built-in excuse to refuse sex.

Today no one can assume anything about your sexual beliefs and standards (your policy). You could believe premarital sex is wrong, or you could believe sex is a form of recreation. You could believe in equal sexual rights, or you could believe that one gender exists for the sexual pleasure of the other. People in our society hold a most amazing, and rather scary, variety of sexual attitudes. Partners will need to bring up the subject of sex before sexual involvement might occur— and let the other person know where they stand. All the experts on STD and acquaintance rape recommend this plan. Our society has too many conflicting messages about sex for people to make any assumptions about another person's sexual intentions. Such suppositions are no more accurate than mind-reading.

Keep another issue in mind as well. Unless you have total sexual nonresponse (don't feel at all interested in sex) when you're touching someone to whom you're attracted, that person will know if you're aroused. Your partner needs to know what that arousal means and how far you will go with it. The confusion over how far a partner wants to go is becoming a very serious matter in the United States. Numerous surveys, for example, show that men who rape acquaintances often believed she meant yes when she said no. *You're living in a society where sexual confusion is the norm, and it's especially important to make sure your messages are clear.* Of course, forced sex is never your fault even if your partner did misread your intentions, because anyone forcing you should stop at the first indication that you are not willing.

The kinds of words the couple use here could be very important. You may be passionately kissing and petting and say, "I don't want to go further." That may not be literally true; you probably do want to, physically. It may be that you don't intend to, that you plan not to, that you believe it is not best. It may help the partner to know that even if your body language suggests that you want to go further, you have decided something else. It sounds like a small thing, but it's critical with some people; the situation is set up in our society for a partner to interpret passion as intention to have intercourse.

Let's say Lauren and Keith are sitting in her living room. They've been kissing and they're beginning to pet with clothes on. Lauren doesn't intend to have intercourse at this time, even though she would like to. She is popular, has dated a lot, and is looking for a long-term relationship. As attracted as she is to Keith, she realizes that she can't go to bed with everyone she dates and be safe.

Lauren: (Sits back on the couch for a moment.) You feel so good. (She smiles.)

Keith: You, too.

Lauren: I need to . . . talk a minute . . . I . . . guess you may be wondering what's going to happen between us. I'm very attracted to you. (She touches his hand, smiles.) I like this, it's great. But I need to let you know how far I intend to go with it. I don't want you to misunderstand what I want to do. . . . (She stops to look for his reaction. He's listening. In fact, his eyes are wide open. So far, so good.) You know what I mean?

Keith: Yeah.

Lauren: I like you a lot and . . . I'd like to keep seeing you. I'd like to see what develops between us. But . . . I've decided I can't . . . go to bed with someone, I can't have sex with someone I'm just dating. I'd have to be . . . steady for quite a while, serious about someone to go that far. (She looks at him, concerned.) I hope you understand what I'm saying.

What Keith says at this point could go any of several ways. A mature person who is capable of seeing another person's viewpoint would listen and understand what she's saying. He might make a few persuasive remarks, but would finally accept her limits or say that he is not interested in waiting and wants a different kind of relationship. But an immature person—of whom there are many—might really have trouble understanding another person's sexual rights. People who try to manipulate others with lines are immature— like a child who is lying to get a treat. For various reasons, there are more Americans who want instant gratification than ever before. People who want what they want when they want it lack what we call the ability to postpone gratification. Demanding sex from another person—or becoming furious when they refuse—is immature and sometimes dangerous.

Let's see how Lauren could react to Keith:

Lauren: (Continues to finish her policy statement.) I'd like to keep dating you, I really like you. I love to kiss and...do what we're doing tonight. But I'll have to stop when it comes to keeping our clothes on. That kind of helps me to keep it under control, you know what I mean?

Keith: Yeah, I think so . . . (frowns).

Lauren: So that's what I'd like to have happen between us, to keep dating and not to go further than we have tonight. (She looks at him, concerned about his reaction, smiles.) Would that be . . . would you agree to have a relationship like that for a while?

Here Lauren has done two things:

1. She's told him her policy. She could be even more explicit, so that there is no room for misunderstanding: Exactly what is she willing to do and exactly where does she want to stop?

2. She's asked him for the kind of relationship she wants to have right now, and asked him whether he agrees. Experts in the field of human relations urge partners to specify exactly what they want to do in a relationship and ask the other person to agree to it out loud. They should not assume that their understandings are clear. Once you agree you have a kind of unwritten contract.

Modern sex educators often point out that a couple can find safe ways to become sexually satisfied—ways that do not entail any sexual risk. What you are willing to do can become part of your policy statement.

Adults Can Be Abstinent

Abstinence deserves a place here as one totally safe option to sexual involvement. And teenagers are not the only ones who need some skills to remain abstinent under sexual pressure. Suppose you are beginning to date someone you really like, but you do not want to take any sexual risks. You decide you're going to limit your sexual involvement until you have a more serious relationship. Then you go out with this new person and at a critical moment when you need to explain, you feel at a total loss for words. What prevents you from being comfortable explaining your decision to the new partner? It's usually one of the following reasons:

1. *You're afraid the other person will think you're immature or unsophisticated.* This results in your feeling somewhat embarrassed, if not humiliated. Such a feeling usually happens to young people who are sexually inexperienced. Mature adults are not susceptible to this kind of pressure. If adults have suffered from premature sexual involvement, they may even envy the sexually inexperienced!

2. *You're afraid you'll lose the person* before you're even off to a good start. This usually happens when (a) you're not confident enough to explain your feelings and let the other person decide if he or she can cope with your limits; (b) you feel pressure to please others rather than yourself—that is, you have trouble being assertive; or (c) you know full well the other person is not going to wait until you feel comfortable with sexual involvement; he or she will look for someone else. If a partner demands that you become involved very quickly, this could mean that he or she is not capable of considering your feelings. This is hardly a good start for a relationship.

3. *You think you'll be sexually frustrated.* This may be true, depending upon whether you have other sexual outlets with masturbation or with non-penetrative (less risky) activities. The best advice for this problem is knowing that (a) abstinence is not permanent unless you decide it is, and (b) while it may not seem so at the time, millions of humans who have been in that situation have lived through it.

It is not unreasonable for you to ask a new adult partner to wait through a somewhat frustrating time while you want to be abstinent. Both partners have a right to leave, of course. But one of the wisdoms acquired with age is that, when you're doing what someone else wants rather than what you think is really important, it may be a warning. It suggests there's something off balance in the relationship.

The history of how we value virginity and abstinence is a colorful one with rapid swings in every direction. Gradually during the revolt against the antisexual Victorians of the nineteenth century, sexual restraint became linked with having hang-ups. The influence of psychoanalysis and other therapies gave birth to the idea that the well-adjusted adult has no "unhealthy" inhibitions about being sexually active. Sophistication became linked to sexual experience. Predictably, in the sixties a new seduction line was added: "What's your *problem?*" A more urbane kind of sexual pressure was possible now, by making people feel that there must be something wrong with them if they were not open to sexual activity.

Not only that—sexual intercourse has become totally separated from parenthood and linked with intense pleasure. "To a large extent, the concept of *pro*creation has been replaced with a concept of *re*creation."[4] Edwin Yoder writes:

> *Long before they are emotionally mature enough to deal with the powerful stirrings of the glands, children today will often have formed a confused and shallow but essentially mechanical view of sexuality, severed from the affections that go to make a good and lasting bond.*[5]

Billboards, jokes and the media—all seem to be telling you that you deserve sex without consequences. But keep your right to sexual freedom in perspective. There have only been about twenty years in human history when people were told that they could be sexual without *seeming* to pay any price—roughly, the sixties (when the birth control pill was invented) and the seventies. When AIDS was diagnosed in the early eighties, this unprecedented interlude was over. In the past couple of years, an open respect for abstinence has become downright trendy. The fear of AIDS has created a swing back to emphasizing restraint. Not only is virginity getting a bit of support among high school students, but temporary celibacy (abstinence) is also being seen as an option by a number of mature adults.

Vigilantes Out to Clean Up Sex Ed

A major obstacle to good sex education in our country is that it has become politicized. Some religious or parent groups scrutinize sex educators ruthlessly and try to force them into one of two extreme categories: those who support virginity and those who support condoms. Sex educators who support condom education may be cast as libertines who are totally against abstinence; and those who support abstinence may be seen as religious, antisexual fanatics who can only parrot "Just say no."

We should provide sex education both for the abstinent and for the sexually active. It is irrational to ignore the simple reality that sexually active people may not revert to abstinence. And abstinent people may need support and information to help them to be comfortable and confident about their position. In our present epidemic of serious STDs, every person who is not in a committed, monogamous relationship needs to at least consider the advantages of abstinence. Rather than perceiving a period of abstinence as a negative, immature, or neurotic decision, some people view it as a positive time of stepping back, thinking before deciding, giving themselves a breather and avoiding risks.

Since the media have done an excellent job of portraying sexual involvement in a positive manner, I am going to debunk some of the myths about postponing sexual involvement. I'll start with advantages for adolescents, but even if you're very experienced, you may be surprised to find some logical reasons that apply to adults. First, if you are looking for emotional intimacy and want to rid yourself of loneliness, you can have a significant, or even a very close, relationship with another person without penetrative sexual activities. After all, strangers can have casual sex and intimates can be platonic. Second, the powerful emotions resulting from sexual involvement can distract you from major developmental tasks you need to complete before moving on. Young people preparing for careers may especially need to direct their energy to other important activities. The emotions of beginning and ending a romance are very disruptive to concentration. In recent years we have even seen *children* who are upsetting themselves over pretend-love relationships. One of my evening students, a teacher, told me it's not unusual for her to see one of her fourth grade girls sobbing because her boyfriend broke up with her!

What is happening to these little children? They need to be playing and studying. In a different way, a high school or college student can be tremendously distracted by the deep emotions elicited in sexual and/or love relationships—the lack of concentration during the up times, the depression and anxiety during the down times. When you're being educated for a career, you should not feel compelled to enter a sexual relationship just because you're an adult now. You might ponder a line from AA: "This is where you're meant to be and this is what you're meant to be doing."

Third, many people who become sexually involved too soon complain of painful feelings that were really not worth it. They might feel shock and a loss of trust when they discover that this person, so intimate with their bodies, has never called back. Or this person has talked about their sexual behavior or perhaps even bragged about or made fun of it. Other disturbing emotions can result, ranging from embarrassment to anger and humiliation. Fears that the other person was infected with an STD are notorious for occurring the morning after but being conspicuously absent just before sex.

Shana, for example, has been on an emotional roller-coaster. She believes that she shouldn't go to bed with just anyone, but if she's dated someone for a few weeks and really likes him, she does. She even insists on a condom. But for a while she's been having a big let-down every few weeks when she or the guy she's dating decide to stop seeing the other. Shana has had just enough time by then to fantasize about how this person could be the one. She has even confided personal secrets to this person, assuming the information will be confidential. When they stop dating, they are so physically involved that it's very painful to lose this intimacy, especially when this virtual stranger has lied or done something else to bring home to Shana the fact that this guy isn't worth it. Looking back over her last few months, she wonders if the frustration of abstinence wouldn't have been better than these unpredictable emotional swings. If Shana does decide to have a relationship, at least she knows that there are ways to obtain sexual satisfaction without penetration or other sexually risky activities.

Any time you enter into any relationship not based on mutual respect you run the risk of being hurt. When that relationship is sexual you can also feel used. Adolescents are unusually vulnerable to this kind of reaction. Teenage girls tend to find sex less pleasurable than boys, and far more girls than boys believe they are in love with their sex partners.[6] These young women often appear to be having sex to please someone they care about, while the meaning of sexual intercourse to boys or young men is often quite different. Boys are more likely to see sex as scoring—a competitive accomplishment rather than a relationship.

A fourth reason to support abstinence has to do with health. These reasons go beyond the risk of disease, covered in Chapter 5. You may also want to be a parent someday. Sex educator Marion Howard, Ph.D., states the case very well:[7] She writes that "the best way for young people to protect their ability to conceive and bear a child or to father a child is to begin to have sexual intercourse as close to the time they wish to begin having children as possible." Young women who have multiple sex partners are at greater risk for STDs and cervical cancer. The health of infants can be endangered by the diseases young mothers contract. Multiple sex partners can also harm the fertility of young men who want to be fathers someday.

Howard writes in simple concepts that hit home. If a pregnancy occurs at a young age, she explains, there is a greater likelihood that the mother will have complications or die in childbirth. In addition, the child of a very young mother is more likely to have health problems or other lifelong handicapping conditions, such as mental retardation.

Abstinence is important for junior high and high school students because we want adolescents to grow to an adulthood when they are capable of having "meaningful, intimate relationships that include a satisfying sexual life."[8] Howard's program "Postponing Sexual Involvement" has surprised educators all over the country, because her simple, straightforward approach has actually taught thousands to use restraint thought to be old-fashioned ten years ago.

Temporary Abstinence for the Adult

Sexually experienced adults usually assume that they will become intimate in the natural course of dating someone. Without religious or community sanctions to restrict you, you can have several sex partners in a relatively short time. Dwight Lee Wolter writes about how he made a strong commitment to stop getting sexually involved with anyone for a while. He reflected that he had spent his entire life reacting to women—what they will do or say or when they will come or go. He had essentially given them great power and control over his life. He felt he had spent years feeling angry and abandoned each time a relationship ended. He was suspicious of his feeling that life was always either being spent in pursuit of, in the midst of, or recovering from, a sexual relationship.[9] One day Wolter had the insight that underneath these painful emotional swings he was desperately searching for the approval of women. He was making choices. He concluded one night that as painful as loneliness was, it did not compare to the loneliness he had experienced with women:

> *I knew that with a vow of temporary sexual abstinence I was leaving many relationship power-plays behind me. I thought I was also avoiding intimate relationships. I discovered that I was only avoiding sexual ones. As a result of celibacy, my relationships with women actually became more intimate. With sex out of the picture, I was able to relax as the tension of expectations, role-playing, seduction, and maneuvering melted away.*

He found that if he took his time, he didn't get into relationships so soon that he had to spend all his energy figuring out how to get out of them. The time he remained celibate gave him a chance to know himself and to find other ways to experience excitement, adventure, love, and mystery in his relationships with women. . . . "Abstinence makes the heart grow fonder," he concluded.

The Acid Test

We know people don't run their sex lives by some set of rules, because passion is powerful. And some of the most rational people have sometimes done something sexual that was risky and on which they reflect back with great relief that they were not hurt. But if you're really letting your higher brain get through when you're thinking of becoming sexually involved, you should ask yourself the following questions:

__ **1.** Am I ready to assume full responsibility for consistently using birth control?

__ **2.** If I do not believe in abortion, am I in a position to assume responsibility for providing for and nurturing a child? Am I financially and emotionally prepared for pregnancy, and parenthood for 18 years? Does the other person oppose my views on abortion, so that if a pregnancy resulted both of us would be thrown into a further crisis?

__ **3.** Am I prepared to take the risk of contracting a sexually transmitted disease, knowing that no current barrier method guarantees safety?

__ **4.** Am I prepared to ask my partner to go with me to be tested for HIV/AIDS before engaging in risky sexual practices? (See Chapter 5 and Appendix for ways to get an accurate HIV test.)

__ **5.** Am I willing to divert the emotional energy required in this relationship from other important concerns such as school, a new career, or my child who's just been through divorce?

__ **6.** If I decide to be abstinent, am I comfortable that my decision is a mature one, self-protective and assertive, best for me, and a way of caring for myself?

The Confidence of Your Beliefs

If you are a virgin, or have decided to become abstinent again, it's important to have confidence that you are right. There is no rational reason that anyone can use to put you down, insult you, or embarrass you because of your decision. If you believe this, you will be much more comfortable about the whole subject. And remember, postponing something does not mean you're giving it up. You hope to actually be enhancing your sexual relationship someday.

Arousal and Guilt

Some partners feel uncomfortable resisting pressure, as if they were somehow depriving their companions. "Naughty me for not giving you what you want." I was once on a call-in radio show when a fourteen-year-old girl phoned to ask for advice. Her problem was saying no. The moderator asked why she had sex with this young man and she replied, "I didn't want to hurt his *feelings.*" American women pick up the idea that they shouldn't deprive men, and men may feel confused about staying in a relationship without intercourse because there are no adult models to show adult males how to date without sexual intercourse. Our models tell us that since abstinence is frustrating, real grown-ups of course have sex when they're dating. But this viewpoint means one thing to the couple who has been going out steadily for a year, and quite another to the popular person who has three dates every week.

Sharing a Partner

"I caught my girlfriend cheating on me," said my student casually, "and we had a big argument, but it's patched up now." In these days when young couples almost expect to have sexual intercourse relatively soon after they begin to date, I think we underreact to cheating on someone. If you have a committed relationship and your partner has sexual intercourse with someone else, I recommend that you take it very seriously. Intercourse is not the same as having a date or kissing. True, some people think of intercourse as just a human act that can be perceived as casual or serious, but you're better off to view it as a major decision. Especially if you want to have a permanent, committed relationship someday, viewing sex with an easygoing, blasé attitude won't work. Also, that person who cheated on you may have exposed you to every disease of every partner that other person has ever had. Regardless of what other so-called "modern" views you may hear, I advise you not to ever share a partner; expect more of yourself and the other person.

How Men Can Respond to Pressure

Some college counselors report a surprising number of young men who are worried about sexual pressure from women. It is so unacceptable to refuse a woman that these men become anxious and concerned about their sexuality. They wonder if there is something wrong with them because they don't want to go as fast as their partners do. Some gays and lesbians may have similar concerns but are often afraid to ask for professional help.

We need to rethink what it means to be a man. A real man can use his brain and not always his body. A real man can turn down a fight and should be complimented for having the strength to solve a problem nonviolently. A real man can decide whether it's wise to have sex with a particular partner. He may find his sex drive hard to ignore, but he can base his sexual decisions on the reality of the situation and not on the advice of his locker room pals or his buddies at work. Men are truly among the brainwashed. They are not only brainwashed to assume that they can't turn down sex, but they are brainwashed to believe they have no self-control. *Up to half of American adolescents agree that rape is justified if a female "gets a male too aroused" and stops.* To show further how confused we are on this subject, surveys that ask, "Have you ever forced intercourse on someone?" find higher rates of agreement than surveys that ask, "Have you ever raped someone?" The implication is that force is to be expected, but it really isn't rape unless it's a rare case involving special circumstances.

Many men do not realize what a tremendous put-down it is to portray men as sexually out of control. Our culture is so enamored of the image of the muscle-bound hunk that the idea of a male being barely under control seems somehow complimentary. "Real potent guys" can barely hold back. But it is not complimentary. Men with a high sex drive may be proud of their sexual capacity, but to stress that it's barely under control implies that men are not trustworthy and can't be held responsible. This concept shores up the belief that men should lay careful battle plans to overpower the opponent, women. More experienced men are sometimes better able to think of assertive responses to risky sexual propositions. What are some of their suggestions for how to resist pressure?

She: I don't want to have sex with you—I want to make love to you.
He: I know, and I'm attracted to you, you know I am. But I'm just not ready to get that involved right now.

She: Come on, honey. Are you afraid or something?
He: It's much more than that. It's an important decision. This is really . . . great, but I like to control my own decisions.

She: Do you have some kind of sexual problem?
He: I hope you don't start questioning my manhood just because I want to make my own choices.

She: I'm on the pill, honey, you don't need to use a condom.
He: It's just my policy, I won't have sex without one.

Saving Face in the Locker Room

Males need to learn how to assert themselves when other males pressure them to brag about sexual conquests. Teenage males, especially, may boast about their conquests, but some men don't outgrow this tendency. Gayle M. Stringer and Deanna Rants-Rodriguez suggest ways that guys can change how they respond to the "locker room bragging"[10]

A says: Who was that fox?
B replies: Carmen was the girl I was with.
A asks: Did you score?

B replies: Hey, I wasn't playing a game.
A says: Was she any good?
B replies: We always have a great time. or: She's a lot of fun to be with.
A says: What's the matter, doesn't sex turn you on?
B replies: Sure, it turns me on, but my private life is my own business and
it's not something I want to talk about with everybody.

How can men say no, or say that they want to postpone sex? In class role-plays, college men being pressured by a woman often go on trying to resist for a few minutes, like this:

Male: No, you're pressuring me.

Female: Come on, what's bothering you?

Male: Nothing, I just need to wait.

Female: What's your problem, honey?

Male: Well, I . . . have another girlfriend.

The man says the last line, which could also read, "I'm moving out of town," when he runs out of excuses. One young man turned to me after the woman had pressured him for about one minute and said, "Help!" It is so rare for a man to turn down sex that there just is no vocabulary for it. Or, at least, nothing that could be said in front of other males. I've noticed that the older the man who role-plays, the better job he generally does in giving the partner good reasons. One reason could be partly that their self-esteem doesn't depend so much on what their buddies think. Teenage males tend to be terrified of their peers' disapproval. But a real man does not give others that much power over him. A mature man does not conduct his sex life for the approval of his buddies.

The Double Bind

Sometimes confusing messages put men into what we call a *double bind*. This is a term for being in a conflict with another person but not being able to talk to her to resolve it.[11] The double bind can be seen in the proverbial joke about the mother who bought her son two shirts. He wore one shirt. When she saw him in it, she protested, "What's the matter, you didn't like the other shirt?" Since he couldn't wear two shirts, he was in a bind. Because he couldn't talk to his mom to resolve the issue, he was in a *double* bind. Just being aroused and having to use your brain to be sensible is, in itself, a bind. But if you're aroused and need to talk about something *and* believe you cannot speak about it, that is a *double* bind.

There are other sexual situations that put a person into a double bind. For example, an incestuous parent is supposedly there to protect the very child he is exploiting. This is a double bind for the child, who cannot ask for protection from his own parent. A partner who gives come-on messages to another and then says no puts the other into a bind. Which one does she mean?

If a woman seems to be saying no and a man feels she really means yes, he should get out of this double bind by asking, not by pushing:

A: No, I can't, don't. . . .

B: (Pulls back and looks at her.) I keep feeling that you want to keep going, but you keep saying no. I don't want to do anything you really don't want to do.

A: Well, I . . . I don't want you to think less of me.

B: I won't think less of you whatever you do, but I need to know what you really mean. It's tough to stop now, but I need to know what you want.

If you have the skills to be sexually assertive and believe you can get your feelings across to the other person, you can avoid a number of sexual double binds.

How Women Can Respond to Pressure

There's no reason women and men could not say essentially the same things in responding to pressure. Most suggestions of what to say apply to either sex. True, women don't have to defend their femininity as often as men may defend their manhood, and men can't specifically say they re afraid of getting pregnant. But the basic reasons to refuse or postpone are the same.

Here are some possible replies to some of the pressure lines described earlier in this chapter:

He: Don't worry, I'm sterile.
She: I know you want to make me feel safer, but . . . well, I'm just not comfortable having sex without a condom. I've known a few people who were more fertile than they thought.

He: You can't get pregnant the first time.
She: Hey, where did you get your sex education? People can get pregnant any time they have intercourse, even if it's just for one second.

He: Don't worry, I'll pull out.
She: I know you want to reassure me, but people can get pregnant that way, even without ejaculation.

Or, if you're on the pill: I'm not comfortable with the idea of having intercourse without a condom on all the time.

A: If you don't have sex, I'll find someone who will.

B: I'm really shocked that you would threaten me like this. I need you to really listen and consider my feelings. (or): I can't believe you are making a threat like this. I'm furious that you would treat lovemaking like some kind of a job, as if anyone will do.

A: I'm a virgin and I've only got six months to live.

B: I certainly hope you can find someone to give you the experience you think you need. But I have to do what is best for me. Sex is not a charity donation.

A: You're such a bitch.

B: It's hard to believe you want to make love to me and you think calling names will put me in the mood. I need to leave now. (Remember, a name caller is more likely to be an acquaintance rapist.)

A: Are you frigid?

B: I can't believe you really mean that. I really get turned off when you put me down. (or): I resent being called names just because I tell you what I want to do with my body. (or): I really get mad when you question my sexuality just because I want to make my own choices about going to bed.

A: Our relationship will grow stronger.

B: I know you really would like to get more involved right now. But I need to wait. And lots of people have had their relationship grow stronger without intercourse.

A: I don't want to do anything. I just want to lie next to you.

B: The way we're attracted to each other, I don't think that would be a good idea. As much as I care about you, I'd better not spend the night.

A: If you loved me, you would.

B: You know I care a lot about you. But I feel very pressured when you try to get me to do something I'm not ready for. It s not fair to me. Please consider my feelings.

A: You're not considering my feelings—you are selfish.

B: Too bad I can't do what we both want, but we both want different things this time.

A: You're my girlfriend—it's your obligation.

B: If you think sex is an obligation, we need to think about this relationship right now. (Watch out for any such talk—it is very common in abusers and rapists. At best, it's an irrational comment by an immature person.)

A: I'll say I love you after we do it.

B: Bye now. (There is no way to deal with a person who would say such a thing. If you stay in a relationship with such a person, lots of luck. Try the counseling advice in the Appendix.)

A: You're a *virgin?* Get serious!

B: I am serious. And it's something I have strong feelings about, too.

Your Body Is Not Debatable

Some people believe that to resist sexual pressure you have to come up with reasons. So it follows, if your partner gives a good reason, you'd better have a good answer for every reason, or else. Suppose you are not a very wordy person and you're out with someone who puts a lot of verbal pressure on you. You don't have to engage in a debate. *You don't have to say anything except "I don't want to."* It's your body. It's not as if he's asking you to lend him an object that you own. Your body is not an object.

A: Come on, you know we'll use protection. Come on, it's natural.

B: No, I've decided it's not a good idea. No.

A: But why? Come on, what's your problem? You know I'm safe.

B: I don't want to.

A: But . . . there's no reason. I don't understand you!

B: That is a reason. I don't want to. I like you a lot, but I just want to have a good time and stop at this point.

That's what you have to get straight: If you don't want to, (or if you don't intend to), that is your reason. Or you can even say, *"I don't know exactly why, really, but I just feel this way."* Imagine if someone wanted you to try to eat a food you did not want.

A: Come on, please try it, you'll like this kind of vegetable.

B: No, I don't want any.

A: But . . . why not? What s your problem? It's delicious.

B: Well, the color, maybe slightly the odor, the experience might not agree with my digestion.

A: That's no reason. The color is great. Please, please have some. You haven't given a good reason.

B: Well, let me try to explain. . . . I guess it's because I feel . . . etc., etc.

You wouldn't do that—you'd just say, "I don't want any." *You do not owe anybody an explanation when you say no to sex, either.* Yes, it may be harder to turn down sex than Brussels sprouts. If you want to offer explanations, if you think it's appropriate to the situation, then do so. But you don't *have* to explain. Take a deep breath and remember your rights.

How to Deal with Being Rejected

A big fear people may not even be totally aware of when they're being assertive is the fear of being rejected. "If I come on strong, she might just tell me to get lost." Or, "If I say what I want, I'll hurt his feelings and he won't like me anymore." Or, "If I tell her I want to wait, she'll accuse me of being weak or something terrible." The bottom line is, you *must* be able to tolerate the idea of being rejected in order to be assertive. For that reason, Chapter 3 discusses the right mental attitude. A dialogue runs inside your head all the time. Here's how that fear of rejection comes up in your self-talk:

She: Come on, Bill, I want you so much.

He: I'm attracted to you, too. I'd just like to wait awhile. I'm not ready to go that far. (I hope she doesn't put me down for that. Is that a frown on her face?)

She: But . . . I'm not asking you to do anything you don't want to, but don't you want me? (Is there something wrong with me? God, I'd like to have sex with him. Maybe I can talk him into it.)

He: Yes, I want you . . . but not right now. It's too soon. (I wonder if she'll tell everyone.)

She: You know, you're downright insulting. Am I ugly or something?

He: I don't mean to insult you. I'm very attracted to you, and I'd like to get to know you better. (Damn, she's going to push me on this. I feel so uncomfortable. It's embarrassing, but I'm doing the right thing.)

No one likes rejection. But you can live through it if you don't make it a catastrophe. Remember, you're worth protecting and you're worth taking care of. A respectful person listens to you and cares about your feelings. Anyone who would reject you just because you don't take care of his or her sexual needs is making a totally self-centered statement.

The very act of coming up with your own answers will help you learn ways to talk back to sexual pressure. It will also help you to become aware when someone tries to manipulate you, so that you develop the protective part of yourself that looks out for you. Even if you become sexually involved with an honest and fair person, that person's interest may not be the same as yours. Or that person might be impulsive at a time when you need to stop. You must always check with your own feelings and be able to talk about them.

Talking About Your Sexual Policy

You talk about your sexual policy when you tell anyone else how you feel about anything sexual. Do you want to be casual or committed? Do you want to get sexually involved soon, or wait a little while or a long time? Do you want to be involved with someone who is basically cautious, or fun-loving and carefree? In these times of sexual confusion, it's good to bring conversations around to what you, or others, think about sex. You could do this in a social group, or alone with a partner.

The purpose of this exercise is to help you get comfortable telling someone else about your sexual policy if the need should arise. Although in real life you'd probably not dot every i and cross every t, writing this assignment will help you to cover some of the toughest sexual issues so that you'll be better prepared.

Imagine that you are sitting around with someone to whom you are attracted. You want to know what he or she thinks about getting sexually involved. Answer the following:

1. How could you break the ice and bring the subject around to the topic of what you think about sex? (Hint: what could you bring up from the media? Or events in your school, college, or work place?) Write how you would begin this policy conversation: "I'd say. . . . "

2. Imagine that you are interested in dating someone and the question of how you feel about sex arises. Knowing that you really care what this person thinks of you and want this person to be attracted to you, how would you describe your sexual policy? Put it in your own words, and don't write what you think you *should* say.

3. What might be questions you'd want to ask the other person? Try to imagine yourself asking these questions. Think about how you might weave these questions into a discussion so they will be easier to talk about— rather the way you might ask people how they feel about politics or religion.

4. If you told your sexual policy to your best friend and felt you would not be judged in any way, what would you say?

5. How did your answers to numbers 2 and 4 differ? What made the difference?

6. Someone you would like to date asks what you think about birth control, pregnancy, or abortion. What do you say?

How Would You Answer?

Practice what you would say, in your own words, to reply to the statements below:

"Why not? We both need it."
  You reply:

"We'll use protection, it's okay."
  You reply:

"But I thought you loved me!"
  You reply:

"Are you a child or a woman?"
  You reply:

"Are you a man or a boy?"
  You reply:

"Is something wrong with me, aren't you attracted to me?"
  You reply:

"But I have needs!"
  You reply:

"It s only a natural act, it doesn't mean anything."
  You reply:

"Grow up, little girl."
  You reply:

"Let me show you how much I love you."
  You reply:

"Now you have me all hot and bothered."
  You reply:

" Don't worry, honey. I'm on the pill."
  You reply:

"I know you're a normal guy, and you're attracted to me. What's wrong?"
  You reply:

Notes

1. Sol Gordon, *Seduction Lines Heard 'Round the World and Answers You Can Give* (Buffalo, N.Y.: Prometheus Books, 1987).

2. Research by Susan B. Cochran and Vickie M. Mays, reported in their letter to the editor of the *New England Journal of Medicine* March 15, 1990, 774.

3. Kelly and St. Lawrence, *Behavioral Group Intervention to Teach AIDS Risk Reduction Skills*, 43.

4. Marion Howard, *How To Help Your Teenager Postpone Sexual Involvement*, (New York: Continuum, 1991), 5.

5. Edwin Yoder, "In Sexual Revolution, is Religion a Contra?" *St. Louis Post-Dispatch*, 13 June 1991, 3C.

6. From a survey of 503 teenagers by Roger Starch, reported in *Contemporary Sexuality* 28, no. 7 (1994), 11.

7. Howard, *How to Help Your Teenager Postpone Sexual Involvement*, 3.

8. Howard, *How to Help Your Teenager Postpone Sexual Involvement*, 10.

9. Dwight Lee Wolter, "Sex is not Equal to Intimacy: Using Abstinence to Establish a Balance in Intimate Relationships," *Inside Recovery* 4, no. 4, (August–September 1992): 1.

10. Gayle M. Stringer and Deanna Rants-Rodriguez, *So What's It To Me? Sexual Assault Information for Guys* (Renton, Wash.: King County Rape Relief, 1987), 10.

11. Don Jackson and J. H. Weakland, "Conjoint Family Therapy: Some Considerations on Theory, Technique, and Results," in *Changing Families*, ed. Jay Haley (New York: Grunt & Stratton, 1971), 16.

5

Speaking Up to Avoid
Disease and Pregnancy

Lust makes you stupid.[1]
—SYLVIA (NICOLE HOLLANDER)

We inherit one connection that is absolutely basic: the link between sex and pleasure, between sex and being alive. To avoid sexually transmitted disease (STD), we
have to make a giant mental leap: We also have to connect sex with pain or death.
There is something inherently unnatural about that connection; it goes against our
biological programming. The human race does not seem very proficient at imagining death (or even pregnancy) as an outcome of sexual intercourse.

This chapter will help you learn how you or your partner can use improved
communication to avoid acquiring an STD or becoming pregnant. It is not just for
those who have no STDs at present, since people affected with one can acquire others. That's another mental distortion: the idea that lightning can't strike twice in the
same place.

How Widespread are the STDs?

Table 5.1 shows the major STDs in the United States and their symptoms.

The Centers for Disease Control estimate that the approximate numbers of people affected in the United States are:

45,000 new AIDS cases reported each year

1,000,000 infected with HIV, the virus that causes AIDS

TABLE 5-1 Six Sexually Transmitted Diseases: Some of the Warning Signs*

	Chlamydia	Gonorrhea	Genital Warts	Herpes	Syphilis	AIDS
Cause	Chlamydia trachomatis bacterium	Neisseria gonorrheae bacterium	Human Papilloma virus: HPV	Herpes Simplex Virus Types I and II	Treponema pallidum bacterium	Human immunodeficiency virus: HIV
Symptoms in Women	Usually no symptoms; occasional vaginal discharge. Burning upon urinating. Pain in abdomen. Bleeding between periods	Usually no symptoms; occasional vaginal discharge or painful urination. Bleeding between periods	Single or multiple soft, fleshy growths around anus, vulva, vagina, or urethra. Itching or burning sensation around sex organs	Single or multiple blisters or sores on genitals. Generally painful but disappear without scarring; may reappear	Four stages: 1) painless chancre—red spot later forming a sore; 2) skin rash or mucous patches; 3) latent stage, no symptoms; 4) complications leading to possible death	After initial infections, may be asymptomatic for years. HIV-related illness progresses to symptomatic phase: fatigue, poor appetite, weight loss, diarrhea, night sweats; the last phase is AIDS, in which other infections cannot be resisted by damaged immune system
Symptoms in Men	Usually discharge and painful urination	Usually discharge and painful urination. Some have no symptoms	Itching or burning around sex organs. Single or multiple soft, fleshy growths around anus, penis, or urethra. Painless	Same as for women	Same as for women	Same as for women

When Symptoms Usually Appear	1 to 30 days after exposure	2 to 21 days after exposure.	1 month to 1 year after exposure	1 to 30 days after exposure	3 to 12 weeks after exposure	Months to years after contact. May have no symptoms for years but can still infect others.
Some Potential Consequences if Untreated	You can infect partners. Various inflammations, including pelvic inflammatory disease in women, which can lead to sterility. Sterility in men.	You can infect partners. Various severe complications, including pelvic inflammatory disease in women, which can lead to sterility. Sterility in men.	You can infect partners. May lead to precancerous conditions. Cannot be cured.	You can infect partners. Cannot be cured	You can infect partners. Death. Disease rarely progresses this far today	You can infect partners. HIV infection progresses more rapidly to AIDS (Acquired Immune Deficiency Syndrome) without treatment. Death
Some Potential Consequences to Infants Born to Infected Mothers	Eye infections and pneumonia	Severe eye infections.	Growth could obstruct birth canal	Infection of infant. Caesarean delivery may be advised	Death, bone deformities, nerve disorders	Some infants will be infected and go through same stages as above

*Other symptoms may occur—seek medical advice, to be certain.

1,100,000 new cases of gonorrhea ("clap")

3,000,000 new cases of trichomoniasis

500,000 new cases of genital herpes (40,000,000 affected totally)

120,000 new cases of syphilis

100,000–200,000 new cases of Hepatitis B

4,000,000 new cases of urethritis and chlamydia

750,000 new cases of genital warts (HPV)

1,000,000 new cases of nonspecific, pelvic inflammatory conditions that result in over 100,000 cases of infertility every year

These are only some of the major diseases. To show you how some of this translates into your odds of being exposed, consider that one in six sexually active people in the United States is infected with genital herpes.[2] The current estimate for the number of people infected with HIV is one in 250.[3] However, among the people in whom you are sexually interested, the odds might be much different. That 250 includes grandparents and children. Sexually active people would have a higher rate of infection.

One symptom of an STD is a burning sensation when urinating, but the absence of such signs does not necessarily indicate health. The experience of Bill and Lisa, two university students who had been dating for several months, shows how disease may be silent in one partner and show up only when her partner becomes infected.

> *Bill began to have difficulties with painful urination, but despite repeated treatment with antibiotics, the symptoms persisted. His disease, chlamydia, now the most widespread bacterial STD in the United States, can cause sterility and be passed on to newborns.*
>
> *Unaware that she carried chlamydia, Lisa was not treated until Bill had failed several times to get rid of it. He received several rounds of antibiotics from a couple of doctors before he recovered. Now Lisa and Bill are both fine, but they could have prevented the disease.*

Many STDs go undetected because the victims don't notice their symptoms or there are no noticeable symptoms. Note that complications such as pelvic inflammatory disease, sterility, or danger to the infants of pregnant women, in addition to potentially fatal infections, may result from undetected or untreated STDs. Less than half of the women with gonorrhea observe any symptoms. We now believe that herpes has infected people who are unaware of it. The sores of syphilis may be painless and disappear although the person is still infected. The partner with whom you're considering having intercourse could even be a carrier of more than one disease and not know it. Researchers estimate that one person could possibly acquire as many as five STDs in one act of intercourse. Unlikely? Yes. But this claim dramatizes the possibilities and destroys the myth that people with one STD cannot get another one. Most STDs are curable. Seek medical advice if you or your partner has any of the symptoms on pages 80 and 81. If you have questions about STDs, call the following Centers for Disease Control hotlines: STD hotline: 1-800-227-8922; AIDS hotline: 1-800-342-AIDS. (See Appendix for further hot lines.)

Attraction

I can make you an absolute, iron-clad guarantee: Anyone to whom you are sexually attracted will seem totally disease-free. Not only that, but I can assure you that if you become sexually involved and use condoms, after a while—with no test or further reassurances—it will seem perfectly natural and safe to stop using protection because you "know" your partner. However, your lover could be just as infected as when you were careful. Nothing has changed except your belief. In moments of passion, that person seems, if not decent and honorable, at least irresistibly magnetic and safe. Becoming further involved, letting your body feel everything it wants to, seems wonderful, beautiful, delicious, and the only reality.

In the sixties and seventies, for the first time in human history, the pill appeared to free millions of people from worry about pregnancy. For the first time, life seemed to promise that everyone could at last enjoy sex to the fullest without any undesirable consequences. But even then, STDs were taking their toll. Long before AIDS, millions suffered from the other STDs. It has just taken more openness as the years pass for us to face the rising STD rate. STD has been a secret between doctor and patient, or a secret shared with no one, or not even recognized as a disease by the person harboring it.

Finding Your Risk Triggers

Maggie loves desserts. The times she most wants dessert are when she finishes dinner or comes home very hungry in the afternoon. These events trigger her sweet tooth, and her desire usually centers on chocolate, but, in a pinch, she'll settle for anything sweet. If she plans a fruit dessert at those times, however, and keeps her favorite goodies out of the house, she eats very little dessert but is still satisfied.

I used to help my clients to quit smoking. We spent a lot of time listing their triggers—the situations in which they wanted a cigarette. For some, it was the end of a meal or talking on the phone. Others associated a drink with cigarettes. In order to become nonsmokers, they learned new ways to avoid their old triggers, things that lured them into old habits in an automatic, thoughtless way.

This concept also applies to avoiding STDs. It is very important when breaking a habit to find your triggers. Getting into high-risk situations rather than having low-risk sex is something you can control, just as a person wanting to eat healthy food doesn't hang around by the junk food machine when he's hungry. If you take sexual risks, you need to trace back to discover what kinds of situations support your high-risk behaviors. Does hanging out in bars trigger your making sexual contacts or going home with someone? Do you have fantasies of high-risk behaviors but never fantasize about safer sex? Do you hang out with a gang whose members brag about their sexual conquests and pressure you to tell all?

Among the major triggers for high-risk behavior is taking a mind-altering chemical such as alcohol. If you use chemicals during times when things might get sexual, all the good intentions in the world may not give you good judgment. I know a young woman who has had five STDs. She has several drinks when she's out at night, but she doesn't make the connection that normal inhibition—her normal resistance—is lowered every time she drinks. Many of these chemicals have the same effect; they shut down good judgment. This is one reason so many crimes involve alcohol. If you think you may be in a situation in which you're tempted to have sex, find something nonalcoholic to drink and eliminate any other mind-altering drugs. You want to keep the rational part of your brain in its best working order.

To see whether you have any triggers, fill in the blank with as many actions as you can:

When I ___ I find that I don't protect myself as well as I can from STDs.

When I do not ___ I don't take as many sexual risks.

How many triggers fit those sentences for you? You may want to make a list of your triggers so that they become a reality to you rather than a trancelike stimulus of which you're barely conscious. A trigger can be somewhere you go, something you do, some drug that you take, or certain people you choose. And your age or sexual preference does not matter—anyone can have triggers. For example, John says his triggers are drinking alcohol with a sexually attractive acquaintance and hanging out in bars where people make sexual contacts. Casual sex is taken for granted in many bars. Both of these practices often trigger risky sex for heterosexuals and gay males.

Mother Nature's Plan

Mother Nature does not like to be fooled. She determined thousands of years ago that, really, she had but two goals for you: one was to keep you alive, safe from serious dangers such as being gored by the buffalo, and the other was to get you (or your girlfriend) pregnant. She devised a terrific pair of the rosiest-colored glasses through which you look every time you see your partner. She fixed it so you will never take off those glasses as long as you're passionately attracted to that partner.

Unfortunately, disease is a hitch in nature's plan. We have a sex drive, but we don't have a drive to avoid STDs, because the drive to reproduce tends to overpower any other considerations. We have other built-in protective tendencies, such as disliking bitter foods (which might contain poison) or blinking our eyes when something comes hurtling toward us. But the strong motive for sexual reproduction leaves us with nothing to protect us from disease except one thing: *our brain's ability to plan ahead and project events that have not happened.*

Studies show that at least one-half of single people take major sexual risks. One of the greatest risks is lack of caution with new partners. And many people take a risk after getting to know the person when they stop using condoms.

Part of nature's plan to get people pregnant causes another mental distortion that blocks good judgment. That is called the *personal fable.* It is the belief that "it can't happen to *me.*" *I* can't get pregnant, *I* can't really get a disease, *I* can't die. Even married women who get pregnant for the first time report a certain amazement that it's actually happened to them.

I am taking the chance of scaring you a bit to motivate you to take the problem seriously. But the evidence from smoking and other habit changes is that *just scaring* people is not enough. Too much fear may turn on the denial mechanism so that they shut out any information about dangers. Experts in the field of persuasion advise that if you want to protect your health, high-threat messages won't succeed unless the message is accompanied by a specific plan of action.[4] That's why this book is designed to help you plan what to say.

The tendency to deny unpleasant things is universal. Denial is a mental mechanism that we use to defend ourselves from frightening thoughts; we simply block them out—we deny them. Some people use denial very often, whereas others rationalize, project the blame, or learn to cope in a healthy, direct way with things that scare them. Denial might be needed sometimes to block out things that prevent us from functioning, but, easily overdone, it can cause us trouble if we refuse to see a risky situation. The fact that an invisible disease could be carried unawares by a healthy, attractive person simply boggles the mind.

Three Basics about STDs

If you forgot everything else, three basic principles about STDs are the most vital for you to understand.

1. *Infection almost always gets into your body by direct contact.* Sitting on toilet seats or trying on bathing suits, are not highly risky for exposure to live STD viruses or bacteria. Although pubic lice can be transmitted through towels or sheets and trichomoniasis organisms could possibly live on bathing suits or towels, scientists are doubtful that *most* STD organisms can live long enough in the open air to infect anyone. Sharing drug needles that come right out of one person's bloodstream and go into another's, or receiving an infected blood transfusion (now uncommon due to screening) can carry HIV—the virus that causes AIDS—right into your body. Transmission of STDs typically occurs between the genitals and mucous membranes of body openings (mouth, vagina, or anus). Some diseases are passed when one person's body fluids (such as blood or semen infected with HIV, or fluid from an open herpes lesion) contact another person's cut skin or mucous membranes. Although fever blisters on the mouth do not reveal anything about a person's sexual activities, they are a form of herpes and can be transmitted to the genitals.

2. *Your odds of getting any STD are decreased by proper use of a latex condom.* Using a latex condom correctly and consistently would prevent millions of cases of STD. Because they provide a barrier through which viruses and bacteria apparently cannot travel, latex condoms could save your life or your fertility. But condoms are not a guarantee against infection. Condoms can break. Fluids sometimes escape the condom. You have to be careful to use condoms correctly, and you still have to give consideration to the person's sexual history, if you know it. Keep up-to-date on the latest information about protection by calling resources in the Appendix. It is also advisable to buy condoms before traveling outside the United States, since foreign products are unreliable.

3. *There are only two ways you can be sure that you will not get an STD: Totally avoid risky sexual practices; or, in a committed relationship, be absolutely certain neither you nor your partner is infected with anything.* Penetrative sexual activities—activities in which there is penetration involved—are the riskiest kinds of sex. Where body fluids, particularly semen, blood, and vaginal fluid can enter any cut or other opening in another person's body, there is greater risk of transmission of most STDs.

The Major STDs

You've seen in Table 5.1 on pages 80 and 81 the causes and symptoms of the most common STDs. After reading it, most of us probably want to throw up our hands and say, "Hey, it's in the hands of fate, I can't possibly avoid all that, so why bother?" It's easier, however, if you remember that you can largely control your exposure to STDs by learning a few basic things to say and do. The fact is, you cannot afford to allow your body to be the conduit for viruses or bacteria from everyone who's slept with everyone who's slept with everyone that you've slept with. Figure 5.1 shows you how misleading it can be to have an unprotected sexual relationship with someone whom you believe has had no unhealthy contacts.

Chuck is having sex with Linda, who has had only one relationship before Chuck. Chuck has had only one relationship, with a sexually inexperienced girl in high school. Linda dated Ted and broke up with him. Without the knowledge of Linda, who was completely faithful to Ted, he had dated Anne, who had numerous lovers and had even experimented with intravenous drugs.

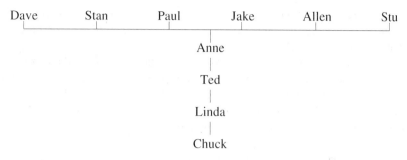

FIGURE 5-1

So you have to get this straight in your mind—STDs can happen to you. Anyone exposed by sexual contact to sufficient bacteria and viruses can acquire an STD. Chapter 3 has shown you some beliefs and rights that you truly need to integrate and believe in to be best able to defend yourself. Long before the moment two people exchange a disease, there are critical times when they could make different choices. At crucial moments, something could be said or done to protect the individual from an annoying, embarrassing, frightening, or even fatal decision.

Of the factors that can influence the partner to be safe, what is *said* is often crucial. Words can powerfully influence what people do, and your words come from the rational part of your brain that is not responsible for leading you into passion. Humans have a unique ability to communicate the most subtle meanings about our desires and needs so we can ask what we want to know about a partner or tell him about ourselves. *On these words may hinge our sexual health, whether we become parents, and maybe even our lives.*

The First Conversation

Before you ever get into a risky passionate embrace with someone and want to go further, you can find out a lot about what kind of disease risk she is. In their first conversations, a person of any age can interview a potential partner. Listen carefully to how she talks about several topics important to you; be alert to signals of safety and danger in what she says. You may be very powerfully attracted to her, but at the same time another part of your mind can assess how safe she might be in a sexual situation. The person who denies danger is the most likely to ignore critical clues from a potential partner.

People wonder, of course, how to bring up the sensitive subject of sex in the first place. How do you start a conversation about sex in general, so that later you could feel more comfortable discussing sex between you two? One of the best openers is to talk about the media: a movie, the newspaper, or TV. That's also a good way to let the other person know what you believe about sex. Discuss what's going on in your country, state, city, or school. Listen carefully to the other person's opinions.

For example, let's take Terry and Marc. They have just met and are powerfully attracted each other. But Terry doesn't want to make a sexual mistake; Terry wants to find out what kind of sexual values Marc has. Terry decides to steer the conversation gradually around to sexual matters—but to sexual things that are far removed from herself and Marc—to get to know Marc better.

Terry: Did you see that ballplayer on the news last night?

Marc: Yeah, I heard he was on drugs big time.

Terry: Well, I saw an article where he said he'd never shoot up because two of his friends had AIDS.

Marc: Huh. Well, ballplayers, aren't they pretty clean?

Terry: They say it's easy to get AIDS from drug needles that people pass around. (Here Terry pauses to see what Marc will add.)

Marc: I don't know, maybe that AIDS stuff is just a big scare. I saw on TV the other night that it's all blown way out of proportion.

Terry: (Decides to come right out and establish the beginning of a safer-sex conversation.) Do you really think so? Well, even the government thinks it's serious. I think people should make sure they're safe.

Marc: Hey, it's not much of a problem for most young people. The rate of infection is really down, I heard.

Terry: I'm surprised you think that, that's not what I read.

Now Terry has been assertive herself and found out that Marc is not well informed. Even though some communities have cut down their AIDS rate by changing sexual practices, there is an alarming increase in AIDS cases among teenagers and young adults. Heterosexuals, gay males, or lesbians, if they use unsafe sexual practices, are all susceptible to AIDS.

Key Phrases to Remember

If you are just beginning to talk to an attractive person, it can help to sprinkle into your conversation a few phrases that show how you feel or asking your date's opinions about sexual risk. You can revise these in your own words.

"I need you to listen to how I feel about. . . ."

"It would be easy to keep going, but I have to talk. . . . "

"I'm attracted to you, but I'm trying to be. . . . "

"I've been thinking about what I would do if we. . . . "

"How do you feel—are we going too fast?"

"I need to get to know someone. . . . "

All Terry has done in the conversation above is listen to Marc's views and bring up issues on which Marc could comment. Here are some other ways to bring up sex in a conversation with a new partner:

"Did you see (name a soap) last night? What did you think of___?" (I can almost guarantee there will be some sexual relationship on which you could comment.)

"Did you see that magazine article. . . . ?"

"Did you see on the news about that woman who. . . . ?"

As you listen to a potential partner talk, ask yourself questions:

1. *Is this person concerned about disease?* Or does she have a nonchalant, care-free attitude based on fun above all? Someone like that can be very attractive but also very dangerous to your health.

2. *Is this person honest in his nonsexual dealings?* Does he try not to hurt other people unnecessarily, or is he inconsiderate of other people? When talking about politics, job, friends, or family, do you hear this person show caring about other people? Or does he take any opportunity for personal gain when no one is looking? These general traits usually carry over to other areas of life.

3. *Is this person considerate of you?* The way you're treated in nonsexual ways probably reflects your partner's basic consideration. If you're always expected to go to the movies that he chooses, for example, or see people that only he likes and never the ones you like; if you're expected to cater to him with no thought for your needs, he probably will also be sexually disrespectful of you.

Does that sound as if you'll have to find a perfect person? What you're look-ing for is not some kind of ideal person who doesn't make mistakes—you're look-ing for someone with whom you could trust your sexual health. It's acceptable for your date to have faults like being messy, late, or too quiet. But certain faults are too important to overlook. The simple truth is, many potential lovers have no con-cern for your welfare, although some of them might seem enormously attractive. You can decide to go ahead and have that fun, or you can decide to use your brain to protect yourself. Yes, you may have to rule out more people from intimacy if you are this particular. But you have only two choices—rule out anyone who seems inconsiderate and who won't protect you, or take a chance, which might be a big chance, of getting an STD, becoming pregnant, or impregnating someone.

Explaining Ahead of Time

It makes protection much easier if you explain ahead of time, before anything passionate happens, how you feel about sexual safety in general. This explanation is basically a policy statement as explained in Chapter 4. But here you're telling not just how far you will go, but what you need for sexual safety. Not that you should stop in the middle of the movie and whisper in her ear, "I'm for safer sex." Just find a good time to steer the conversation around to the topic of sex, see what happens, and find your opportunity to say what you think.

For example, let's say Joe and Kerry are college students out on their fifth date. They are very much attracted to each other, but they have done nothing more than kiss on their last date. Tonight they're sitting on the couch in the dormitory lounge. Joe picks up the student newspaper, glances at it, and puts it down.

Joe: Wow, there's so much about gonorrhea on the campus now.

Kerry: Yeah, it's really in the news.

Joe: They say people can have it and not know it.

Kerry: I know. My friend's brother has had it twice.

Joe: People really need to be careful. But I think everyone hates to talk about those things. (He makes a face.)

Kerry: Yeah. I guess it's hard to—to talk about. (Kerry's obviously going to let him take the lead.)

Joe: I think people should bring the subject up ahead of time and see if they agree.

Kerry: Okay. Well, I see what you're saying. . . .

Joe: I've thought some about what kind of relationship I'd like to have, and how to be careful. Want to know what I think?

Kerry: Yes.

Joe: I think we should talk about exactly how to protect ourselves if we ever make love.

Joe is letting Kerry know where he stands, and he's also listening carefully to Kerry's attitudes. Would she support him in this? Or might Kerry subtly, or directly, try to undermine him?

Don't forget the policy statement in Chapter 4. You can avoid many misunderstandings if you talk about how far you want to go. If your relationship begins to get more passionate and might proceed to risky sex, it's urgent that you talk about any concerns that either of you has, beforehand.

Mentioning Protection without Accusing

If you've discussed your general views about sex in early conversations, you've laid the groundwork for later intimate talks. Your partner knows how you feel about sexual risks. Now you want to narrow down the focus, because presumably you would not stay in this relationship unless you hoped it might develop further. Your talks become progressively detailed and personal, like the funnel in the diagram in Figure 5.2, until you can talk about sex between you.

How to be Nonoffensive

If you let your partner know you are afraid of disease, any mature person would understand that you're just trying to be sensible and protect both of you. But how can you mention protection with the least possible offense, considering your partner's feelings and preserving the relationship that matters to you?

Starters.

It's good to have a few little starters to help yourself approach the things you need to say. It's okay to mention your feelings:

"I need to get more comfortable talking about. . . . "

"I'm not sure I can explain this perfectly, but. . . . "

"It would be easy to go on without saying this. . . . "

"I want to be fair to both of us."

"You know, I see the news and I keep thinking. . . . "

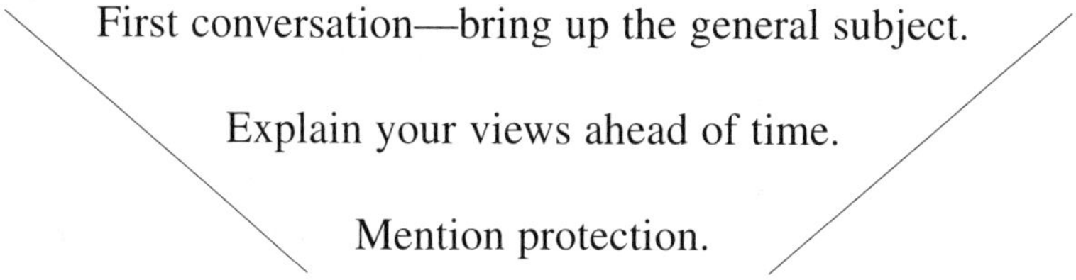

First conversation—bring up the general subject.

Explain your views ahead of time.

Mention protection.

FIGURE 5.2

If you are bringing up protection early in a relationship, you are right. You are cautious and mature about it; you are doing the smartest and most ethical thing.

Men in our society are supposed to have courage. The media show examples of supposedly desirable courage—killing, hitting, driving fast, courting physical danger. How about the courage to speak up? That takes a lot of bravery, and we need to recognize it and admire it. People who speak to their friends about their concerns and say the tough things—I admire those people. Their courage opens an opportunity for others to speak their minds as well:

"I'm really scared about how you might react, but. . . . "

"As embarrassing as it is sometimes, I think someone has to have the nerve to speak up."

"We need to have the guts to talk to each other ahead of time."

Imperfect Talk Is Okay

I'm giving you a lot of material here so that you can absorb various helpful phrases along the way. If you don't put them in this order, if you repeat yourself and stumble a bit, don't worry about it. You're not a robot or an actor. You might even condense all the important things down to two sentences:

"I'm not comfortable doing that."

"If we continue to date, we'll have to _____."

But the more you read and hear about sexual assertiveness, the more it becomes a part of you. In fact, you need to hear yourself say things out loud. If you're reading this on your own, try some practice. Stand in front of the bathroom mirror and *say the things you want to say out loud*. If you need to, take this book with you and go over some of the things you want to be able to say. You could even use a tape recorder in order to hear yourself and begin to integrate that it's really a part of *you* when you talk like this. You may feel foolish talking to the mirror. (Is she kidding?) No, I'm not kidding. Are we discussing something important or not? Studies show that all people can remember better if they practice aloud, whether they're giving a speech or asking for a raise. They also feel more comfortable later, when they really have to speak their part; it's familiar and they've stored it in memory. Of course, if you explore the idea in your own words, so much the better. You will feel much more comfortable being sexually assertive in your own natural speech patterns. The acid test of sexual assertiveness is whether you mean what you say and you say it in a genuine and unaffected way.

Lying Is Common

I knew a woman in her late fifties who was lonely, having lost a child and a husband. She met an attractive man; they dated and went to bed without a condom. Afterward, she said, "You don't have any diseases, do you?" "I have herpes," he replied. "Why didn't you tell me?" she exclaimed. "I always tell people if they ask," he said.

Please don't believe everything a new, attractive person tells you. It is very difficult for many people to admit that they've taken some sexual risks in their past. Even people who are generally honest and caring, when pressed for the precise risk they might have taken, tend to present themselves in the best light. People who want sex with you will be highly motivated to persuade you. Therefore you must proceed as if any new sex partner *could* be infected.

Getting Specific

How can you two start talking about protection? If you pick a time when you aren't sexually aroused you're more likely to be able to set things up ahead and give your partner time to digest what you've said. Let's say Alex and Kelly have been going out together. Kelly has already laid the groundwork by preparing Alex for the conversation about condoms. What happens from here? Kelly chooses a time when they are not involved in a passionate embrace—perhaps earlier in the evening, alone in the kitchen over a snack, and sober.

Kelly: (takes Alex's hand, rubs a thumb across it.) I haven't forgotten what you said last night about . . . wanting to make love.

Alex: (Grins) I haven't, either.

Kelly: You make me feel really great. I guess you can tell, by the way I talked the other day . . . that I think people should talk about protection before they get involved.

Alex: Uh, yeah, I remember.

Kelly: Well, I think all that stuff you read about—about using condoms—is right. I think people should use them, the right way. This is kind of hard to say. . . .

Alex: I hope you don't think that I have any—

Kelly: No. That's what makes it so hard to talk about these things, because it sounds like you're trying to accuse someone else of having a disease. Still, anybody could be carrying something and not know it. We could have been lied to, or we could have been with someone who was a carrier and didn't know it.

Kelly tries to reassure Alex. The most mature people respect their partner's reasoning on this subject, but it's usual to push or persuade in the heat of passion or with the prospect of "scoring." If everyone you date is pushy and pretends to be insulted when you're asking for protection, if they all treat your sexual opinions with disrespect, that doesn't mean you have to put up with it. It just means you've run into lots of people who are immature. You might want to look at why you're picking such people and where you're picking them.

For example, Jan has met five men in bars and discos, which are the only places she thinks she can meet guys. Two of them stood her up occasionally and made fun of her for wanting to postpone having intercourse. The third got so pushy she thought she might be raped, and she did not see him again. The fourth and fifth men wanted sex without emotional commitment. When Jan didn't, they dropped her. Jan's unhealthy reasoning goes something like this: "There must be something wrong with me. Or else there's something wrong with men—they can't be trusted." So she continues looking for the right men in bars. Because of her self-concept ("I'm not a goody-goody") she thinks there's nowhere else to really meet anyone.

A healthier approach might be, "I've been trying to meet people in only one place. While some nice people may go to bars and discos, they are places where alcohol and loud music make conversation almost impossible. Also, only a small proportion of the guys I might meet go to those places. Could I join a health club or political organization or other group where I would meet a different type of person?"

How to Ask for a Condom

We left Kelly and Alex beginning to talk about protection. Now they're at the point where it's time to discuss condoms. Remember, a condom is not foolproof. Going to bed with multiple partners *using* condoms subjects you to higher risk of disease than unprotected sex with one healthy partner. The reason is that condoms sometimes leak or break, and they may fall off if they are not carefully held in place during withdrawal. Even so, Kelly has decided to have sex with Alex and she wants to minimize the possibility of their transmitting diseases. Their conversation might go like this:

Alex: Okay, what do you want to do?

Kelly: Well, I want to use condoms, for one thing. That's about the least couples can do, don't you think?

At this point, Alex may go along with Kelly's plan:

Alex: Okay, I agree. Do you want me to buy them?

Kelly: Okay, or I can. There's one more thing.

Alex: (Laughs.) Okay, what?

Kelly: They have to be latex and have that spermicide on them.

Alex: (Chuckles.) Gosh, you've really got it down pat, Kelly.

Kelly: (grinning) I've been readin' up.

But what if Alex is putting pressure on Kelly not to use condoms? What if the conversation went this way?

Alex: A condom! That's like taking a shower in a raincoat.

Kelly: I'm sorry to hear you feel that way. (I-statement.)

Alex: God, you can't be serious! I can't feel anything that way.

Kelly: I've heard that lots of guys who use condoms felt enough to satisfy them.

Alex: (Now he's in a power struggle and bluffing to see who can win.) Nah, it's not for me.

Kelly: Are you saying, then, that you wouldn't use condoms, no matter what? (Kelly wants to get it clear before making a decision.)

Alex: Yeah.

Kelly: You're saying you'd rather not go to bed with me at all than to use a condom? (Kelly sounds as if it is unbelievable that Alex would say such a thing.)

Alex: (Frustrated by the truth and maturity of Kelly's statement.) You—you don't know what you're talking about! I haven't got anything! (Remember, this anticondom attitude makes Alex more likely to have been exposed to an STD in the past.)

Kelly: You know, Alex, I'm not willing to go to bed with someone who puts my life on the line. If you're not willing to do this simple thing to help us both . . . I guess we're not going to go any further in this relationship.

Alex: You're so selfish!

Kelly: That's merely your opinion. To me, it's caring about myself. I get really mad when you call me names for standing up for myself.

Here Kelly and Alex have arrived at a basic decision point. Remember that self-esteem strengthens people to take care of themselves. Kelly may feel very disappointed right now. She was hopeful and excited about her relationship with Alex. But right now freedom from an STD depends entirely on what's going on inside Kelly's head. If she feels able to tolerate being alone for awhile, it will be easier to reject Alex. If she can really feel angry about his insults, rather than passively tolerate them, it will be easier to reject Alex. *Because what just happened is that Alex insulted Kelly for trying to protect her body and maybe even her life.*

Psychologists teach people not to label others unfairly. Communication experts emphasize tolerance for the values of other people. But sometimes a label is necessary. A conversation about sex is no occasion to tolerate just any old opinion. Some of us have met so many immature and selfish people that we really don't register a simple fact: There's no future in a relationship with a person who won't even use a condom to protect you both. There may be some temporary fun in it, but recognize the amount of risk and weigh it against the fun.

Other Condom Comebacks

A: Just this once?
B: It only takes once.

A: It doesn't feel good to use a condom.
B: I'd feel a lot better.

A: It spoils the mood for me.
B: It puts me in the mood.

A: It takes too long.
B: You'll be turning me on every second.

A: You won't catch anything from me.
B: When a man cares, it's so sexy.

A Quickie Condom Conversation

If you're a person of few words, of course, there's no need for a long discourse on condoms. Probably quite a few first sexual encounters go like this:

A: Got a condom?

B: No.

A: Oh, honey, we've got to use a condom.

B: Maybe next time?

A: No, I really want to use one.

B: Nothing can happen right now.

A: No. Want to go to the drugstore with me?

Better yet, A already has one that she chose because it's the safest and most effective kind of condom.

Condom Realities

A condom, used correctly and consistently, is extremely effective in preventing the transmission of STD. It is safer, but it is not safe. Condom use also has a high, but not perfect, reputation for preventing pregnancy if performed consistently and correctly. However, it would not be fair to portray condoms as risk-free. It's wise to consider the best-case and the worst-case scenarios before you decide. A physician and father phrased it this way in *Newsweek*:

> Abstinence and sexual intercourse with one mutually faithful uninfected partner are the only totally effective prevention strategies. *I am going to tell [my daughters] that condoms give a false sense of security and that having sex is dangerous.* Reducing *the risk is not the same as* eliminating *the risk. . . . There is no safe sex. If the condom breaks, you may die.*[5]

Asking for Birth Control

Asking a partner to use birth control involves the same techniques of assertion as resisting pressure and asking for protection from disease. If you are a woman who is neither on the pill nor using a birth control device, you can check the safety of properly used devices at a local Planned Parenthood or other clinic (See Appendix). But if a man is using condoms to protect you from pregnancy, it's best for you to have a say in what kind of condom is used and how it's used. You should tell him pertinent facts about the pill that you are taking. Each of you has an absolute right to know that you are protected, and how. For example,

Lawanda: I'm glad you bought the condoms. What kind are they?

Rob: They're expensive—they're supposed to be good.

Lawanda: Could I see?

Rob: (Looks slightly embarrassed.) Sure.

Lawanda: (Reading label) Oh, I see they are made of animal skin. I heard that kind aren't as safe because viruses and bacteria might pass through those microscopic holes.

Rob: (Looks crestfallen.) I tried to get good ones.

Lawanda: I know. When we go out for a snack later we could stop by the drug store and exchange them. (She kisses him on the cheek.) Thanks for caring.

Does this sound nervy? She has three choices: Use a kind of condom that has been proved less effective, use the safest kind of condom, or avoid sex for now.

If you are a man who is not in a monogamous, trusting relationship, do not trust just any woman to use the pill carefully. Do you want your future as a father to depend totally upon someone's memory to take a few *pills*? Using condoms properly would reduce your concern about her mistakes. *And* using a condom can assure you of greater protection from disease. Some women lie to men about being on the pill when they are not. Some women have fantasies of marrying a guy someday and, although they are not consciously trying to deceive him, unconsciously take chances on getting pregnant.

Discussing Your Outlook on Abortion

Regardless of your beliefs about abortion, I think you should tell them to any partner before having sex. Unromantic? So is being a parent unexpectedly. Unrealistic? So is pretending everything will be okay. There are two kinds of problems that can arise if you never discuss abortion.

1. If you are a woman who would never have an abortion, you could be under tremendous pressure if you get pregnant and the father wants you to abort. If you are a woman who accepts abortion as an option, what if your partner does not agree, you become pregnant, and your partner decides to explore his legal rights?

2. If you are a man who believes abortion is an option but your partner opposes abortion, you can be a father, and have long-term financial obligations, with even the most casual partner. Or you could oppose abortion and have a woman aborting in a situation in which you want to become a parent.

If you aren't sure how to approach this, how about opening a discussion about articles in the news? There's always some issue about abortion coming up in the newspaper. You can easily find out your partner's views if he or she is honest about them, without even discussing sex between you two.

Some Helpful Phrases About Contraception

"I really need to use condoms even if you're on the pill."

"I think it's important to double up on birth control."

"I feel very uncomfortable when you keep pressuring me to stop using condoms."

"I'm sorry if it's not what you want, but I need to do this."

"It's just a policy of mine to always use condoms."

Time Out! What to Say in the Middle of Things

Jeffrey Kelly and Janet St. Lawrence are two researchers who have taught a lot of people how to have safer sex. The groups they trained to be assertive have drastically reduced rates of HIV infection. One of their best ideas is to role-play how to stop in the middle of sexual activity if something unsafe is about to happen. They say their research groups found this the most difficult, but also the most helpful, role-play, even though it was X-rated. These are some of the kinds of unsafe practices that might start to happen:

> *Anal sex*: It is so highly correlated with HIV infection (the virus that causes AIDS and hepatitis B) that experts simply advise, don't do it. A person having anal sex even once in a year greatly increases his chances of HIV infection. Other STDs could also be transmitted anally.

> *Penetration without protection*: Condoms must be used before penetration begins and continued throughout intercourse.

> *Withdrawal without holding the condom in place*: Condoms may fall off after ejaculation, spilling semen and, with it, viruses or bacteria. Pregnancy can also result from this mistake.

See Appendix for places you can call to ask about high- and low-risk behaviors. Listed on page 224 you'll also find a pamphlet that explains little-known hygiene methods to reduce the chances of an infection. And keep informed about new findings concerning all STDs. National hotlines and other places where you can get information about STDs are listed on page 223 and in the Appendix.

There's no way around it: If you are in a sexual situation with someone who tries risky sexual practices, you have to stop it. If you can do it with your body language, fine; if not, you can say, "No!" and move away or otherwise make sure it can't happen. You don't have time to stop and have a conversation. And remember, a little temporary embarrassment is far better than a major life crisis. I also mention how to stop in the middle of things for those who are having sex unexpectedly with someone new. Responsible professionals in the field of sexuality advise against multiple sex partners, and sex with someone you do not know is obviously highly risky. Every new partner may increase your risk. But realistically, many people engage in casual sex. If you are sexually active, take this moment to imagine that someone is attempting risky sex with you, and picture or hear what you would say and do to protect yourself. Fantasizing is a good method of practicing. Of course, you can easily come up with a simple phrase to stop things when they're getting risky. But it's good to see some time-out statements in writing and to hear them, because your society has never shown them to you:

"Stop. I need to stop."

"Wait. We haven't taken care of . . . ."

"Whoops! We almost forgot the condom."

"No. Remember our talk?"

"No, I have to use condoms."

"No. I feel very strongly about this."

"I won't do that."

"I don't want to."

"Time out!"

What if, all over America, people who need to stop at any point in sexual arousal would hold up their hands in the T sign of sports and say, "Time out!"? (Well, maybe not in the dark.) I can imagine that this might become a good-natured way of stopping in the name of safe sex, as common a phrase as "Get off my back!" or "Give me a break!" It would be okay, and expected, and so socially acceptable that everyone would know what it means.

How to Ask for an STD Test

You may find that this beautiful person before you looks as clean as a whistle. But your higher brain knows he could have an STD. There is no test for any STD that couldn't be reversed by the time the test results are in. That is, if Jenny gets tested on Friday, you and she can read the report that she is disease-free on Tuesday; what did she do on the weekend? And tests for HIV must be taken after a waiting period of several months after the latest risky sex took place in order to be accurate. Trust is still the most vital element in relationships. Mike and Jamie are another couple who have been dating awhile and have already talked generally about what they want to do to protect themselves.

Mike: (Sitting on the couch, he has been kissing Jamie for a half hour.) I want to make love to you, Jamie.

Jamie: (Smiles dreamily.) Me too.

Mike: (Sits back, looks away.) God you are so—you just hit me like a ton of bricks. (Runs his finger down Jamie's face.) I need to talk, though.

Jamie: Okay. (Smiles.)

Mike: All the things you read about—I've promised myself that I'll take the time to talk to a new person that I'm starting to care about. I've been reading that . . . maybe the only way for people to know they're safe . . . to know that someone hasn't, you know, given them something . . . is to take a test. (Grins awkwardly.) This is hard to talk about.

Jamie: I hope you don't think that I—

Mike: No, no, it isn't you, or me. It's just . . . the times, I guess . . . a really nice person could have something and not know it.

Or maybe Jamie objects:

Jamie: Hey, are you saying I have AIDS?

Mike: (Touches Jamie's arm.) No, I'd never say that to someone I like as much as you. It's just . . . nobody knows what the people they were involved with before have done. It's getting so . . . anybody could have anything, I guess. I hate to say it, but how would I even be sure about myself? Will you go with me to get tested?

There are various tests for a number of STDs. As of this writing there are tests for HIV antibodies in the blood. *It is important, even if you are reading the latest book you can find, to call the hotlines and keep informed about the latest kinds of tests for STDs and what they mean.* A new and important finding could occur the day before you call. Do not assume that some kind of clean card carried by anyone has any meaning whatsoever. The only way for a couple to be tested for an STD would be to discuss it together with the medical professional, wait the required number of months with no sexual risk, have the test, receive permission to see each other's test results in the presence of the medical person—*and* totally trust that the partner has not become infected before or since the test was taken. Sometimes HIV, the virus that causes AIDS, can be present in a person's bloodstream, yet not show up on antibody tests for many months after infection. However, at this writing the Centers for Disease Control state that nearly everyone who is infected with HIV will show positive on a test taken three months from the time of infection. However, they recommend waiting a full six months before being tested, with no sexual risk during that time, because there are some really rare cases that take that long to show positive. Cases have been *reported* in which the person required longer than six months to show positive on the test, but the Centers for Disease Control have not been able to *document* those cases so far.[7] Because new information may come in week by week, you should call the CDC hotline to confirm any facts about HIV testing: 1-800-342-AIDS. (See Appendix for sources of the latest STD testing information.)

Most physicians do not offer pre- and post-test counseling when they check for HIV, but most government-sponsored and many private testing sites do provide counseling. It is very important to get counseling with HIV test results.

Anyone being tested for HIV infection should be cautious about revealing information concerning the test, regardless of whether the results are positive or negative. There have been cases of discrimination—even when the individual's test was negative. Individuals should inquire ahead of time about confidentiality, without giving their names, before they even consider disclosing any information about their HIV status.

If You Have Exposed Someone to an STD

Some STDs are reportable and some are not. For example, in most states physicians and private clinics are required to report cases of certain STDs, although names may not always be reported. The testing site will almost always ask you to contact anyone you may have exposed. STD experts feel *it is extremely important that you contact your partner(s) regardless of whether you are asked to do so.* Because so many people can have an STD and show no symptoms, your telling the truth may be the only way your former sex partner can avoid serious problems. Think how you would appreciate knowing if you had been exposed to an STD so that you could obtain medical treatment.

There's no way around just coming out with the truth: "I need to tell you something. I went to the doctor yesterday and she said I have chlamydia. She said that I need to be sure to tell you so you can see a doctor soon." You can go on with the facts or pass on a brochure if you have one. Most people, while unhappy with the news, will be glad you've been fair enough to tell them. If anyone gives you a hard time after you tell, you can always say, "Would you rather I hadn't told you? This was real hard to say, and it didn't do me any good, but I figured it could really help you avoid a lot of heartache. I care about you and your health."

If you're wondering how to talk about an STD under other circumstances, such as telling a potential partner that you have herpes, you could call one of the resources in the Appendix.

Legal Issues

If you have an STD and decide to have any risky sexual contact with another person, you should be aware of the legal implications. Attorney Margaret Davis has written a book called *Lovers, Doctors, and the Law* that details the legal concerns involved in modern sexual relationships.[8]

At this point you may be saying, "Hey, now I know I'm giving up and not worrying about any of it—there's just too much!" Fine, but that doesn't change the reality. A well-informed person who is sexually active in these times has a fairly high chance that an STD will become an issue, whether it's exposing someone else or being exposed. Even in college classes, it's common for as many as 20 percent to have had an STD scare of some kind. *Lovers, Doctors, and the Law* explains the legal responsibilities of partners with and without STDs. There have been a number of court cases in which people who were exposed to an STD without their knowledge have taken ex-lovers to court and won. Ms. Davis recommends that you share your medical history with your lover, including the date and findings of your last medical checkup. In addition, she suggests you share information about any previous lovers who had any symptoms of STDs, and any treatment you have had. This precaution in itself might cause you to limit the number of sex partners you have, because how many people do you want to know such personal information about you?

Davis further encourages readers to discuss their recent sex lives and whether either has had any partners from a high-risk group. Again, the answers may be untrue. But a person who lies about his or her disease risk is taking a legal risk, because that person may be found guilty of a civil or a criminal charge.

Davis recommends that lovers make a physical examination for any STD symptoms a part of their foreplay. (This suggestion has been offered by a number of sex educators.) Should you learn anything about the STD history of another person, you are obliged to keep that information confidential. There is a great deal of prejudice, and in some cases risk of discrimination, involved with certain STDs.

Defend Yourself and Your Partner

It is possible for you to be passionately attracted to someone with one part of yourself and still be a bit suspicious with another part. Look at it like this: Would you buy a car and not ask anything about its functioning? Would you lend money to someone without inquiring about her dependability? Your body is a lot more important than your car or your money—it is irreplaceable. Respect it enough to protect it.

If you become familiar with assertive actions like those described in this chapter, you're well on your way to being able to defend yourself sexually. Have courage. You're worth it. Nobody has a right to risk your health, and you are the only person who can protect it.

How Would You Answer?

Whether or not you are sexually active, you need to learn sexually assertive responses. Respond aloud with an assertive statement to each of the following comments:

   1. "But I don't have any diseases."
      You reply:

2. "I don't like to use condoms."
You reply:

3. "It doesn't matter whether they are latex or not."
You reply:

4. "I'll take care of everything—don't worry."
You reply:

5. "You must not trust me or you'd have sex without a condom."
You reply:

6. "Why do you want to talk about all this beforehand? It ruins the spontaneity."
You reply:

Some retorts:

"I don't think you have any diseases. I'd say this to anyone. I don't discriminate."

"I don't like *not* using condoms."

"Yes, it does matter. Latex condoms are safer."

"No, I want to be in on everything that affects me."

"I could let myself go a lot more if I felt protected."

"Being spontaneous is easier when I feel safe."

"I'm really disappointed that you won't protect us."

"A condom is a way you show you care about me."

"I have to care about myself, too, you know?"

"I know you'll understand if you really care about me."

"Anyone can get an infection. A condom will protect us both."

Is Alcohol a Risk Trigger for You?

(If you're concerned about privacy in your answers, write them on a separate sheet) Answer the following True or False:

__ **1.** I feel more comfortable having sex after I use alcohol or other drugs.

__ **2.** I am more likely to pursue a sexual encounter if I am under the influence of alcohol.

__ **3.** I am more likely to have sex when I am under the influence of alcohol.

__ **4.** I have used alcohol or other drugs and then not remembered what I did.

__ **5.** I have become intoxicated and made sexual advances that I later regretted.

__ **6.** I have become intoxicated, made sexual advances that I later regretted, and engaged in sex that I later regretted.

__ **7.** I have had sex when I was not planning to, because I was drinking.

__ **8.** I do not drink or use other mood-altering chemicals and never have.

__ **9.** I drink upon occasion, but none of the above has ever happened to me.

(After finishing this, turn to pp. 229–230 and see the research from various college classes on the above items.)

Notes

1. Copyright 1989 by Nicole Hollander.
2. American Social Health Association, "Herpes Questions, Answers" (Research Triangle Park, North Carolina), 1994.
3. Centers for Disease Control National AIDS Hotline, January 12, 1995.
4. Sharon Shavitt and Timothy C. Brock, *Persuasion: Psychological Insights and Perspectives* (Boston: Allyn and Bacon, 1994), 229.

5. Robert C. Noble, "There is No Safe Sex," *Newsweek* 1 April 1991, 8.
6. Kelly and St. Lawrence, *Behavioral Group Intervention.*
7. Centers for Disease Control Hotline, January 23, 1995.
8. Margaret Davis, *Lovers, Doctors, and the Law* (New York: Harper and Row, 1988), 22–23.

Part III

How to Cope with Intrusion and Force

6

Resisting Sexual Harassment

> *Power tends to corrupt, and absolute power*
> *corrupts absolutely.—LORD ACTON*

"There was this top-heavy gal who had on this skimpy little top. . . . " A professor who makes statements like this in class may be breaking the law. Expecting people to work or study in the face of continual comments that make fun of their gender is as distasteful as asking someone to tolerate racial put-downs. What powerful people do and say can create a hostile environment that makes concentration impossible. And as unlikely as it sounds, direct sexual propositions from faculty occur with astonishing frequency on college campuses, and even in high schools. A major study of harassment at work finds that at least one woman in five has quit a job, been transferred, been fired, or withdrawn an application for a job because of sexual harassment.[1] Recent surveys of the U.S. Army and the U.S. Navy personnel show such conduct to be a serious problem there as well.[2]

It is cynical to believe that every powerful person is corrupt. But the political axiom of Lord Acton that begins this chapter strikes at the heart of sexual harassment: exploitation of a powerless victim. And although the overwhelming majority of victims are women, men also can be harassed and their careers permanently damaged by employers or professors who demand sex.

What Is Sexual Harassment?

According to the dictionary, *harass* means "to vex, trouble, or annoy continually." Always unwelcome, sexual harassment ranges from unwanted sexual innuendos made at inappropriate times—perhaps even in the guise of humor—to coerced sexual relations:

- Verbal harassment or abuse
- Subtle pressure for sexual activity
- Sexist remarks about a person's clothing, body, or sexual activities
- Leering or ogling of a person's body
- Unnecessary touching, patting, or pinching
- Constant brushing against a person's body
- Demanding sexual favors accompanied by implied or overt threats concerning one's job or student status
- Physical assault

Although most harassment is committed by people with direct power over the victim, coworkers are responsible for some incidents. Recent court cases have found employers—including colleges and universities—liable for incidents and conditions that add up to a chilly climate for women. When working conditions make an employee uncomfortable because of the pressure to put up with sexual remarks, gestures, or other uncomfortable sexual events, this too is sexual harassment. For example, if Marie has to sit beside a nude calendar all day and listen to people comment on the breasts of the woman on the calendar, her employer can be held liable for not having removed the calendar and for allowing a hostile work environment.

Sexual harassment is unique among the various ways that people can exploit each other. Unlike many other forms of sexual exploitation, *the victim has something to lose on a daily basis,* and the harasser usually knows it. In no other situation except that of marital rape could an adult be expected to tolerate the constant presence of a sexual abuser. The advice in this chapter is for anyone facing sexual harassment, male or female.

Can You Pick out the Sexual Harassment?

Circle below the actions that would be considered sexual harassment.

1. Your roommates spread a rumor that the woman down the hall is a lesbian.

2. Two students next to you, along with your professor, frequently ogle a *Playboy* magazine and make comments about the women's bodies while you are waiting for class.

3. Your professor covers your hand with his as you are discussing your paper.

4. The hairdresser at the next station to yours continually talks in front of customers about how gorgeous you are and how he wants you to go out with him.

5. Someone is sending you unwanted, explicitly sexual messages through your computer.

6. Your boss compliments you when you have on a short skirt but says, "Why don't you wear that short red one?" when you have on a longer skirt. He's done this several times.

7. Some of your friends call other people babes, studs, or sluts.

8. In class the math professor often jokes about how "girls" don't like math but they'll have to get used to it.

9. At coffee break your manager suddenly starts telling you his sexual fantasy. Then he says, "Now that I've told you what I fantasize about, you tell me."

10. You wonder if it's an accident because it happens so fast, but your boss brushes your breast occasionally while showing you some procedures on the computer.

All of the above, if unwelcome, are examples of sexual harassment.

Like rape, sexual harassment is usually done in private. This results in the average person not comprehending how seriously upsetting and disruptive these incidents can be. Few people realize that harassment is not just issuing sexual invitations to someone; cruel and degrading incidents can occur. For example, in societies where women are treated with disrespect, it is not unusual for men to demean normal female functions. A few years ago I moderated a panel on harassment; one panelist was a woman suffering from posttraumatic stress disorder. She had been employed by an engineering group and was the lone woman at that work site. On her first day she found a dead rat in her desk drawer. Later she found a tampon with red ink spilled on it made to look like blood. Other similar surprises, along with an employer who refused to take action to protect her, left her shaking at her desk and finally unable to work. Susan Webb, an expert on sexual harassment, once came before a group of company men to conduct a workshop. She describes her welcome: "When I went to the front of the training room, one of the men had taped a tampon, colored with red ink so it looked bloody, to the overhead projector. When I asked him why, he said he'd heard that I was a bitch."[3] Would you have thought that this kind of behavior is so common that by chance I heard of two such incidents? Harassment can rob people of their dignity and often of their ability to work. All of the following are examples of sexual harassment:

Larry, a salesman, needed to sell his product to a woman buyer who made it clear she wanted to go to bed with him. She said she would not buy his goods if he did not respond. He said: "I did it so she'd buy from me, but she was ugly and repulsive."

Marcia's graduate school professor asked her to stay late to work on some papers. He suggested sex. After she refused, he lowered her grades. The dean who supervised him felt Marcia was exaggerating. She became so upset she transferred to another school and lost a semester's credit.

Tanya, a young single mother of three, worked in a bank. Her employer asked her to stay after work for some extra projects. At first he merely told her how nice she looked. She tried to ignore him. The next time she had to stay late, he put his arm around her waist and tried to kiss her. She pushed him away with a joke. But the next week he called her at home and said she'd better improve her attitude. When she still didn't go along, he asked to have her transferred.

Leslie, a teenager, worked part-time in a small print shop. One day the boss and another employee wrestled her to the floor in the back room and tickled her. They were laughing, although she was screaming for them to stop. Later the other employee apologized, but the boss said she was making a big deal—it was all in fun.

What Is Not Harassment?

Some men are nervous because their behavior with women at work may be misinterpreted. It is unlikely that a person would falsely accuse another of sexual harassment—the accuser usually has little to gain and a lot to lose. But it is a serious matter to accuse someone of an illegal activity that can harm his career. There is much confusion over what constitutes harassment. We need to define our terms carefully.

Having been raised in an affectionate family, I can understand how someone could make a physical gesture with no intention of offending. I often touch friends on the arm, hug them when trying to reassure them about something, or welcome them with an embrace when they return from vacation. But touchers of both sexes need to be especially alert to the signals of people they touch. Does the touched person flinch? Try to move away? If so, these are indications that the touching is unwelcome.

What can a well-meaning person do to avoid unintentional sexual harassment? Susan Strauss recommends an easy way to determine if your comments and behaviors are wanted or unwanted.[4] People of any age or either gender should ask themselves the following:

1. Would I want my comments and/or behaviors to appear in the newspaper or on TV so that my family and friends would know about them?

2. Is this something I would say or do if my mother or father, girlfriend or boyfriend, sister or brother, wife or husband were present?

3. Is this something I would want someone else to say or do to my mother or father, girlfriend or boyfriend, sister or brother, wife or husband?

4. Is this something I would say or do if the other person's significant other (wife, husband, boyfriend, girlfriend) were present?

5. Is there a difference in power between me and the other person? (Am I that person's teacher, supervisor, or employer, or do I have power over that person for some other reason? Examples: size, social status, etc.)

Some people say that this risk of being falsely accused is the price men have to pay for what they have done throughout the centuries. But I do not like the idea of inherited guilt. If an individual man respects women, his attitude is a powerful asset to society, to women, and to men. Although we don't inherit guilt, we do inherit responsibility; it is the duty of everyone to speak up against the underlying attitudes that support the sexual sickness of our society. Chapter 10 will address those solutions. Here the discussion focuses on methods to prevent harassment or stop it in its initial stages.

The Price Society Pays

Sexual harassment causes the loss of millions of dollars to American industry. After surveying 20,000 federal employees, the Merit Systems Protection Board estimated the cost of harassment to be $267 million over a 2-year period, resulting from job turnover, stress, absenteeism, and reduced productivity.[5] Private industry also pays a high price. *Working Woman* magazine published a now famous survey showing that almost 90 percent of the Fortune 500 companies have received sexual harassment complaints, over a third have been hit with a lawsuit, and nearly a fourth have been repeatedly sued.[6] More recent reports have consistently disclosed the fact that in workplaces across the country, at least one in two women and up to 15 percent of men claim to have experienced sexual harassment.[7] Surveys show that the typical incident for a female involves an unmarried woman and an older, usually married, man. The typical incident reported by a man is an act by a younger, divorced or single woman or by another man. The 15 percent finding about men is probably an exaggeration, because when details about the incident are given, it is learned that the men often welcomed the woman's behavior. Men surveyed tend to view sexual overtures from women at work as mutual, whereas women more often view male overtures as unwelcome.[8] Harassment is, by definition, unwelcome. Women in nontraditional jobs such as coal mining, law enforcement, and surgery report a shocking number of harassment incidents, including rape.

Sexual harassment is degrading, often frightening, and sometimes physically violent. It often takes place over a long period of time. This kind of sexual pressure produces an inestimable loss of productivity and damage to careers in colleges and universities. Hundreds of documented cases exist in which students have had their grades lowered, been forced to change their majors, changed colleges, or switched jobs or even fields, all because they could not stop a pattern of sexual harassment.[9] On college and university campuses, the most reliable studies indicate that up to 70 percent of female students have experienced some form of sexual harassment, including sexist remarks in class, unwanted touching, or outright propositions from their professors.[10]

Students or employees may happily plan their college or work careers and then face with shocked disbelief the fact that they're being subjected to sexual blackmail. Harassment frequently causes profound consequences, including such physical symptoms as gastrointestinal problems or severe headaches that often require a doctor's care. Some people, forced to remain under this unbearable tension, may begin to use alcohol or other drugs to excess. Psychiatric disorders, including post-traumatic stress disorder and serious depression, can also result. Not only are near-ly one-half of harassed people discharged or forced to resign if they do not give in, but often they can't recover financially because they have difficulty getting letters of recommendation or they fear telling prospective employers what happened to them.

Victims of harassment may find it extraordinarily difficult to adjust later, espe-cially because the myths of our society suggest that females create their own sexu-al problems.[11] One reason sexual harassment causes such severe stress is that—as in all sexual exploitation—this victim-blaming clouds the issue for the victim. In this confused society, perpetrators may genuinely believe that the victim is exag-gerating her complaints. Especially if the charges involve being forced to tolerate "a little good-natured teasing" or "mere" sexual comments with no propositions, other workers may call the harassed person a troublemaker. They may further harass the victim and accuse her of being oversensitive and humorless. Victims often search in vain for something they have done or seductive clothes they have worn that may have caused the incidents; or they may try to excuse the perpetrator because "I don't think he meant anything by it."

Women are supposed to be "nice," and are somehow supposed to defend them-selves without coming on strong. Femininity is equated with being passive; an assertive woman is strange and disturbing, a bitch. So women are damned if they assert themselves and victimized if they don't. Even professional women feel pres-sure not to be too assertive; better to respond to offenses with sweetness and com-posure lest they be placed in the bitch category. Voltaire described this distorted sense of blame: "This animal is evil; when attacked, it defends itself."

The Stages of Sexual Harassment

The sexual harasser often begins by testing the potential victim with looks or flir-tatious comments. But some go so far as to sexually assault an employee or student with no preliminaries. There is no way to predict precisely how harassment will begin. As we shall see, in this as in many kinds of sexual exploitation, alcohol is often involved.

Assertive Coping Skills in Dealing with the Harasser

A person who is being sexually harassed is caught in a bind: saying "Stop!" to someone with power is risky. There is no simple solution. The most common and least effective means of handling sexual harassment is to ignore it.[12] There is evi-dence that assertiveness can often improve the situation. It must be done thought-fully, and gauged to fit the level of harassment. Once again, people with high self-esteem tend to recognize disrespectful treatment and are inclined to assert themselves against harassment. If yours is a situation where assertiveness would help, you must believe that you deserve respect. You must believe that no one has a right to make you uncomfortable with unwanted sexual behavior. If in your childhood you were frequently treated with disrespect, screamed at, put down, or otherwise abused, you may feel confused about who caused the harassment.

Even if you are sexually harassed, you probably want to keep your job or stay in your class. All studies show that victims (students or employers) are *very reluctant* to bring incidents to the attention of the organization. But unless they do, this offense can continue unabated. Many employers or school officials think they have no harassment problems because no one complains. Most campuses and employers address sexual harassment complaints informally. The first step in bringing the incident to the organization's attention is rarely an official complaint. Experts urge that you use informal means to begin your complaint, such as going to an affirmative action director, a women's center, an ombudsperson, a human resources officer, a trusted professor, supervisor, or other mentor. Usually you will need advice from some knowledgeable person.

Although you may fantasize about telling off this abuser in no uncertain terms, realistically you may need to think ahead and plan before you act, preferably with good advice from a professional. Most harassment complaints are resolved before they reach the court. Legal remedies against harassment require emotional energy, time, and money; they result in physical as well as mental stress. Avoid them if you can.

What Does She Mean?

The person who wants to cope with harassment has to do a bit of self-evaluation. As I've mentioned at several points in this book, many men read friendly messages from women as sexual. Every group of sex offenders from obscene phone callers to acquaintance rapists shows confusion about this issue. *But misreading women's intentions shows up even in surveys of normal men.*[13] The entire culture aims to convince men that women are oversexed and always available. You cannot be responsible for somebody else's misinterpretation. If you have made your dislike of the harassment clear, the harasser is always responsible if it continues.

Learning a New Professionalism

Harassment in the workplace has been around a long time. Documented cases of sexual harassment occurred in the eighteenth century among housemaids in Boston and "mill girls" in Philadelphia. But because it was taken for granted that someone could abuse power and demand sexual favors, it was not even given a name until 1976. People who suffered "it" endured the unspeakable. Women of my great-grandmother's generation had no name for it when the plantation owner pressured them. Today most workers still have not learned how to leave behind the old, sexist ways of behaving. Men and women need to learn new reactions to each other. It is inappropriate to tease someone about his race or his age; it is equally inappropriate to remark about someone's sexuality at work or school.

Professionally Pleasant Versus Friendly

We Americans consider friendliness a desirable quality and a social advantage. We enjoy being casual and do not require the restraint that is considered good manners in many cultures. Certainly we would not want our employers or professors to think us unnecessarily aloof. Good working relationships go more smoothly when everyone is pleasant. It's fun to look forward to an agreeable day at work or school. But workers and students need to learn a precise line between a *pleasant attitude* appropriate to their role and the kind of *friendliness* that could be perceived as sexual openness by a male in American society. In our hypersexual climate you can best defend yourself if you have some techniques to raise your consciousness. You'll feel more comfortable if you're aware of these issues. You could do a little reversal in your mind to check out your behavior. Let's say you are a heterosexual female. Do you react to your boss with the same attitude as if he were a woman? If you are a gay male, and you have a male employer, do you react to him with the same neutrality as if he were a female? That is, reverse the genders and test whether your behavior communicates sexual overtones:

Employer: That's an *awful cute* dress you have on, Marla. (Winks.)

Marla: Gee, thanks. You like it? (She smiles, knowing it's a sexual compliment. She looks at her employer for a moment and stops work. In the view of the hopeful employer, she responds much the same as she would to a male friend or boyfriend. But Marla does not intend to imply any sexual openness; she's just responding to a man-to-woman compliment.)

That compliment could come from a well-meaning employer, although experts nowadays advise employers to remain impersonal. Compliments on a nice dress are fine—without the wink. Such sexual comments or gestures happen all the time. But she doesn't know what meaning her employer intends to convey. How could she know that he misperceived her response as a come-on? One option would have been for Marla to respond as if her mother or a casual acquaintance had complimented her:

Marla: (Pleasantly, looking up for a moment.) Thanks. (Goes back to her work.)

If you're concerned about how well you stay in your role, ask for some feedback from trusted friends or co-workers. Try to establish that fine line between professionally pleasant and friendly. And sometimes there is a further line, and a very thin one, between friendly and flirtatious or seductive. This advice is not intended to suggest that a victim causes her own harassment—it is to help people give clear messages in case it would help clarify their intentions to confused people. Remember, many harassers will ignore your message anyway.

Friendly Versus Seductive

That line is even more difficult to draw. The comment made by Marla's employer, and the wink, were flirtatious. Of course, it's impossible to ignore someone's gender. But a lot of semiflirtatious behavior goes on in the office or school. It can be fun, and it's harmless—as long as there's no misunderstanding of your intentions. But in the face of this serious national problem, experts advise that, when in doubt, everyone should learn how to be businesslike at work. Flirting may be harmless if the recipient interprets your meaning correctly, but are you willing to stake your job or school success on that?

The Pressure to "Smooth It Over"

One common way a person tries to repel the advances of someone in power is to try to smooth it over. A minority of women are flattered by sexual overtures from supervisors and play along, hoping to get something out of the harasser. Most women are very uncomfortable and simply try to remain pleasant in hopes that nothing harmful will happen. Smoothing it over (by continuing to be just as friendly after the harassment) usually does not work; often the harasser regards it as a positive response or even a come-on. Remember, thousands of people distort the sexual meaning of other people's behavior. With such people you might try to be as aware as possible of your body language. You cannot cause them to harass you, but you can try to be as clear as possible since they're already confused. When you're trying to patch up an argument with a loved and trusted person, you can operate very differently from the actions you need to take against a sexual harasser.

Getting Your Professionalism Across

There are some flirtatious people who are not hard-core harassers. They are often looking for the least signal of interest from you. There are only a few harassers who perceive the other person accurately, but it's worth a try to check your business behavior. If you would be more comfortable learning a few basic rules to help convey businesslike intentions, try these guidelines:

1. Evaluate your eye contact. You know what flirting is. You know how you speak to someone about business. Look the harasser in the eye, but pretend it's your banker or your physician.

2. Perfect the professional smile. Think of how you smile at a sales clerk when you are shopping, or how you smile at someone who helps you in the doctor's office. This smile is not necessarily insincere, just different. Now think of how you smile at someone to whom you're sexually attracted. A smile is often misinterpreted. Even if you're not ready to be assertive, consider very carefully before you smile immediately after an incident of harassment. If you were telling a child to stop being rude, you would not smile or the child would receive a double message.

3. Evaluate the sexiness or business message expressed by your clothes. Remember, illegal sexual activities are never caused by the victim. You cannot cause your own rape and you cannot cause your own harassment. You have a perfect *right* to dress in any way you want that is inside the law or company regulations. *But you are living in a society that is confused about your sexual availability.* The latest fashions are often perceived by men to be highly exciting and seductive. There may be some other kinds of clothes—more modest, more professional—that you could enjoy wearing at school or work.

Your clothes cannot possibly cause anyone to commit a crime against you. I can think of only one kind of sexual exploitation over which your clothing could have even the slightest effect, and that is when co-workers or students are providing a sexually pressuring climate around you. The logic goes like this: A person *knows* when he is forcing sexual intercourse on you, he *knows* when he's threatening to discharge you for withholding sex, he *knows* when he is touching your body without your consent. But if he wants to flirt with you or talk sexy to his coworkers in your presence, he may think your clothing constitutes permission. It clearly does not, and you're absolutely right if you refuse to accept any responsibility for the behavior of your coworkers or a flirtatious person at school. However, it's worth considering that small factor to make sure your message clearly indicates that you are in a professional or a student role. You may be more comfortable feeling that you're aware of what you're doing.

These suggestions are not intended to blame employees or students who are harassed. We have blamed victims for too long. Harassment by its very definition is *unwelcome*. However, if you worked among people who believed stealing money was okay, I'd tell you not to wear your billfold on your hip. Stealing is not right, it's not fair, and the thieves should be held responsible. But if you want to help yourself you have to recognize the sickness of your society's attitudes and try to protect yourself from being victimized by them.

How to Reward Or Punish the Harasser

Another way you might consider using to stop a harasser cold is to *reward businesslike behavior* but *do not respond* to even mildly flirtatious or sexually related behavior. You may also be rewarding others for harassment if you laugh at their sexually harassing words or behavior. Watch for what Caroline rewards and punishes in a conversation with her new boss:

Caroline: When did you want me to do these papers, then?

Employer: (Grins suggestively.) Maybe we could *stay late*, huh, Caroline?

(Caroline acts as if she does not hear, and busies herself with some things on her desk. To some harassers, this is a negative response. The implication is, "I won't respond to that." She will try this once but ignoring will not be a repeated pattern.)

In a few seconds, he turns to her again.

Employer: These should be done by noon tomorrow.

Caroline: (Pleasantly) Okay. I'll get the other folders. (Her implication is, "Now you're acting appropriately and I'll respond.")

Caroline is not cool all the time. She just responds positively when she's treated in a way that is suitable for their relationship. When someone flirts or behaves in any way unbusinesslike, she doesn't answer instantly if she can delay briefly or look away, or she makes it seem that she can't believe he really did say such a thing. This pattern of response is called "shaping," and we do it all the time—it's one way people learn what our limits are. It's not the same as tolerating repeated unwelcome behavior. It's an experiment to see if the person can be frozen out at the beginning, an option for mild and borderline situations.

You may be able to set limits and make yourself clear at the beginning. If harassment occurs anyway, that fact does not mean it was your fault. We're talking about setting limits just as a teacher might with a child who is too loud or too aggressive. Students can also use this shaping technique. Let's say a professor Smith has invited Ms. Santoya into his office to discuss her paper.

Professor: Rayna, this is an excellent paper. I thought you were special, and you are.

Ms. Santoya: (Does not smile but looks interested in his opinion about her paper.) Thank you. I'm glad you thought my paper was good.

Professor: You're quite a fascinating young lady.

Ms. Santoya: (Ignores the last remark and returns to the only appropriate subject.) Did you have any criticisms? I'd like to improve my writing style.

First, when the professor began to get personal, she did not smile. But she said the socially appropriate thing—what she would say in any business or professional transaction. Secondly, when the professor started telling her she was fascinating, she moved the conversation straight back to her school goals.

This technique involves two basic strategies:

1. Reward positive nonsexual comments, act as if they are professional, and respond professionally. This will make you worry less about being unfriendly to powerful people. You are pleasant if they are appropriate.

2. Ignore or defuse personal comments by remarking on the business at hand.

Resist Flattery

Our society is set up so that powerful men are often attractive to women—even if the women are beautiful and the men are not. Power is said to be an aphrodisiac. But powerful people are in a position to misuse their authority rather easily. Tenured college professors who have senior status in their departments are thought to be more likely to sexually harass students.[14] Younger, less experienced women are more likely to be flattered by the admiration of their professors or employers. The professor is often delighted with a younger, uncritical partner and thrives on being looked up to. If you are being sought out and treated as if you are quite wonderful in a situation like this, beware. There are professors who have a long history of sleeping with students after treating them as if they're the only women in the world. And every year they have a new crop of young women from which to select. In *The Lecherous Professor*,[15] the authors uncover the myths that help college professors rationalize sexual involvement with students. Some of these myths are:

1. College women are so beautiful that no man should be expected to resist.
2. College women dress in provocative ways that ensnare men.
3. College women are basically hedonistic and promiscuous anyway.
4. College women need male professors to guide the process of their maturing.
5. Like Pygmalion, the college professor can give vitality and liveliness to these unformed young creatures.
6. The students are consenting adults, and as such freely choose this form of sexual involvement.

The authors comment about the falsity of myth number 6:

> *People who promote the consenting adult myth seldom mention that true consent demands full equality and full disclosure. Students lack not only power and equality; they are also frequent victims of professors' distortions of truth. A student may understand and agree to limits in her relationship with a professor, but faculty Casanovas usually forget to inform the woman that she is only one in a long procession of "consenters."*

These affairs with faculty, after they break up, are often devastating to the self-esteem of the woman.

Folksy Little Maneuvers

If someone is doing something illegal to you, why not consider using any skills at your command? Much as I'm a stickler for the honest and straightforward approach, there are times to think of something creative and indirect to back off a person who is committing an illegal act against you. The following anecdotes have impressed me:

One retort, called in on a radio show on which I appeared, was suggested by a woman who used it when her boss made a pass at her:

We've got this great working relationship and I think you're terrific, and if I did anything to give you the impression that I would be unprofessional with you, just let me know.

She felt this allowed him to keep his dignity after he made a pass.

Another woman says in a businesslike voice, "No, Mr. Adams, I've got two unbreakable rules in my life: no romances with coworkers and no romances with married men. I'll see you at the meeting tomorrow."

Another option is advice from Miss Manners on what to do when someone pats your bottom uninvited:[16] "Fanny patters of any age are treated the same. One screams and then, when everybody's attention is drawn, explains, 'You startled me!'" This could be applied to times when a person is touched in certain other places as well.

Another unique idea involves prevention. You may want to perfect the skill of dropping a warning while you are engaging in a social conversation. This technique can put others on the alert that you are aware of fair treatment issues, or it can raise their own awareness. For example, you could say to a new coworker, "I really think I'm going to like this new job. I love the work. We have a neat health care package, and we've got strong sexual harassment regulations. Seems like the company is very progressive, don't you think?" A student could say, "My parents told me things have really changed since they went to college. Now we have computers to do the research for us, and sexual harassment regulations, and all kinds of progressive things."

When the Harasser Persists

But what if the harasser will not be deflected, defused, or ignored? If Marla's professor persists, like this . . .

Professor: Why do you keep ignoring me? (Takes her hand.)

Here the victim is at a decision point. She wants a good grade, a good recommendation, or a good job. Nevertheless, most experts say that now she needs to be direct:

Marla: (Removing her hand) I'm not ignoring you, Dr. Smith, I just don't want you to do that. (or): I'm trying to keep this a professional relationship, Dr. Smith. (or a very naive rejoinder): Gosh, I'm your student, Dr. Smith.

Suppose a high school coach asks a student to pose in a jockstrap. (I have known these photography-seduction techniques to be imposed upon both males and females, by both male and female harassers.)

Coach: Say, Eric, you know what might be nice? You have a great body, and it might look good to have some shots of you (opens the drawer of the desk, holds up a jockstrap) in one of these, maybe.

Eric: (Taken by surprise, wants to give himself a moment.) I'm not sure I know what you mean, Coach.

Coach: Oh, just put on one of these and we'll take your picture, just for fun.

Eric: Oh, no, *I—I'd feel very uncomfortable doing that.* (or): That's not for me.

Note that he makes an I-statement. A potential victim may not be able to think of anything to say to a proposition, but for some situations you can fall back on the good old I-statement, "I'd feel very uncomfortable doing that." You could say the same thing when your professor or employer invites you somewhere inappropriate to your role, or when any suggestion is made that results in your feeling ill-at-ease. Of course, telling someone you are uncomfortable is a civilized statement that you would only consider making to a nonviolent person. If force is being used, you are usually wasting your time to appeal to the other person's concern about your feelings. Get out of there if you possibly can.

A common tactic used by a professor or employer is to ask very personal questions. Let's imagine that you were not prepared the first time this happened, and you've already answered a few questions that seemed unsuitable. After reading this, you decide you are going to draw the lines of your role more carefully. You could handle it like this:

Professor: What do you and your boyfriend do? Are you . . . intimate with him?

You: Oh! I'd feel very uncomfortable sharing that with one of my *teachers.*

Professor: What for? I care about you.

You: Could I ask you to explain that exam question from yesterday?

This student is sticking to business. She's ignoring the sexual overtones to see whether the professor will give up.

Learn to change the subject. Some hard-core harassers won't allow it, but you can often fend off a tentative harasser with these kinds of remarks. Of course, it takes experience sometimes to be able to banter easily. Practice in front of the mirror. Ask a friend to role-play it with you: "You be Dr. Klein and I'll. . . . "

Coworker Harassment

Employers are legally liable if their employees are sexually harassed by their coworkers. What if a coworker continually makes sexual remarks and you're embarrassed and angry about it? This kind of teasing often falls into the illegal category despite the fact that a person in power is not directly involved:

Coworker: Why don't you just lean over his desk and give him a good look? That'll make him give you a raise.

One option is:

Sheryl: Dan, I am getting really sick of your sexual remarks. This is a *professional* relationship, and sex has no place in it.

Making a Joke

It's difficult for most people to think of a joke as a response to harassment, but some people are artists at turning an insult into a joke. For example, Elissa Clarke tells of a steelworker whose male coworkers howled like dogs when women first showed up on the job. So she brought a box of dog biscuits and tossed one at the men every time they howled.[17]

You might find a way to joke that stops harassment. But you need to be aware that the harasser may already think it's a joke. If you ever decide to make an official complaint, you will need to demonstrate that from the very beginning, *you did not like the harassment*. So if you're good at joking turnoffs, consider using them only for low-level harassment and make sure they work. If the harassment doesn't stop, the joke may be encouraging it.

Avoid Being Alone with the Harasser

Try to avoid being alone with people who are giving you any of the signals of beginning harassment. If a harasser maneuvers you to be alone with him, you could say:

You: I can't stop by your office today—I'll pick it up after your lecture. (or): Sorry, I can't stay late—have to leave on time today. (or take a friend with you.)

Keeping a Record

If you experience even one episode of harassment, you should keep a private, written record of all harassing incidents, and of any complaints you lodge against the harasser, school, or company. For each instance, make a complete record:

1. Where the incident occurred.
2. The date and time of occurrence.
3. What happened.
4. What was said.
5. How you felt.
6. The names of any witnesses or others who have been harassed by this person or at this company or institution.

You may also want to consider two additional steps. Employees have access to their personnel records in some states. You may want to check your personnel file and keep copies of positive evaluations if you can. Better yet, get a copy of good evaluations when they are given and keep them for your future use. Sometimes they are removed in retaliation for your resisting sexual harassment.

Some authors suggest that you carry a hidden tape recorder into any discussions with someone who has sexually harassed you. A tape recording made in this manner probably is inadmissible in some courts. But its legal use is not the reason someone would carry a hidden recorder. It can back up an informal complaint or a formal complaint that stays within the organization or grievance process. One expert on sexual harassment tells me that Susan Sarandon used a tape recorder in exactly the right way in the film *The Client*. The idea is that if you've got the goods on the harasser, the company will be far more interested in settling the complaint.[18] A playback of such a recording to a campus or company ombudsperson could have a powerful effect and could get action fast on informal resolution. For example, the harasser could be seriously disciplined. Carrying a hidden recorder may be illegal in a few states; you need to check that out first.

Arranging a Talk

Suppose you have tried everything you know besides complaining directly to the harasser or higher-ups. To your disappointment, the harassment continues. You could consider arranging a talk and telling the offender your reactions and what you want. For example, let's say Lou works under the supervision of Rachel, who has repeatedly tried to get him alone where she rubs up against him and tries to kiss him. Lately, since he's avoided all of these situations, she's been assigning him an impossible amount of extra work and behaving in a rude and hostile manner. Lou feels he just can't go on like this. He sees she is not going to let up. The situation is unbearable. This job is very important to him. He makes an appointment to talk with her.

Lou: Rachel, you know, I'm really worried about something, and I need to tell you. Over the last few weeks when you've tried to kiss me and touch me, I haven't responded. Now I notice you've been giving me more work and acting really angry at me. (Here he describes what happened.) This has me so worried that I have not slept at night more than a few hours for weeks. I've even had some medical problems. (Here he describes the effect the harassment is having on him.)

Rachel interrupts: You're imagining things, Lou.

Lou: (Here he says what he wants to happen.) Well, I want to tell you how it seems to me. I want you to stop trying to kiss me or touch me. I want to be able to do my job and have a good working relationship with everybody here. I think you and I can have a good working relationship.

Talks like this are one option that may stop the problem before it goes further. An advantage of a talk is that it's still less formal than the next steps you could take. One disadvantage compared to writing a letter is that there's no record of the conversation unless you tape-record it. It will probably not seem as official as a letter, but that could be a benefit as well.

Writing a Letter

Another method of dealing with harassment is the idea of Mary Rowe, an assistant to the president of the Massachusetts Institute of Technology.[19] This technique involves writing a letter to the harasser. Before you do this, try to get the advice of a trusted and experienced person, often a campus ombudsperson or director of the women's center. Rowe advises that the letter include the same three parts as the personal talk above:

1. Describe what happened:

> *"You've asked me out four times."*
> *"You keep mentioning sex with me."*
> *"You've made jokes about my body."*

2. Describe how you feel:

> *"My stomach is in knots all day."*
> *"I can't sleep over this."*
> *"Since then I've had constant headaches."*
> *"I'm so humiliated I want to hide."*

3. Describe what you would like to happen:

"I want to be strictly professional."
"I want you to stop making any sexual remarks to me."
"I want you to treat me like a student."

This action results in some advantages: You have a record, you have taken your own power rather than feeling helpless, and you have proof that you made an active effort to stop the harassment. It is best, Rowe advises, if someone accompanies you when you deliver the letter.

There are also some disadvantages in the letter-writing technique. Lois Vander Waerdt, an attorney and sexual harassment expert, advises that such a letter lets the institution off the hook and makes the target of the harassment responsible for solving the problem herself. The letter could also limit a plaintiff's court case. "If the institutional grapevine gives good marks to the campus or employer for resolving sexual harassment issues, complaining through internal channels is a much more effective means of addressing sexual harassment and getting it stopped."[20] Vander Waerdt points out that harassers usually approach multiple targets; writing a letter only to the harasser won't help anyone else that the harasser approaches and it does not let the organization know officially about the harassment.

Seeking Emotional Support

If you are the victim of sexual harassment, you need someone to talk to besides the official who receives your complaint; it's important for you to get support from people you trust with the whole story and be able to express all your feelings. It's a shock and a terrific burden to face injustice on a daily basis. But in your anger and fright, don't go spreading accusations around indiscriminately, or you may be accused of slander. Talk to professionals or trusted people. In confiding, you may also find others whose ordeals corroborate your own. Most harassers approach more than one person, and have a modus operandi, or typical pattern. Networking with other victims can give you important information and strengthen your case.

Other Options Before Taking Legal Action

You may go to your supervisor, Affirmative Action officer, your adviser or counselor, or your union representative with this problem if you have not been able to resolve it yourself. The appropriate person on a campus could be called an ombudsperson or a designated sexual harassment adviser. Most colleges and employers have specified people to whom you can complain, and who know the internal procedures for addressing sexual harassment. The law requires the employer or campus to *act reasonably*. This duty may mean taking action without your permission, and "reasonably" may *not* mean keeping your identity confidential. If you complain, ask about these two things. Take your documentation with you. You don't have to memorize it if you can glance at your notes. Again, stress the three points: This is what happened, this is how I'm feeling, this is what I want to happen.

Legal Remedies

Despite the anguish that sexual harassment continues to cause, we have made progress. Title IX prohibits discrimination in education at any institution receiving federal funds. Title VII of the Civil Rights Act of 1964 prohibits discrimination in employment on the basis of race, color, religion, national origin, and sex.

But this is not to say that legal action is easy or that it will be the best thing for you. As with rape, the victim sometimes has to undergo distressing mistreatment. One employer defense is to hire a private investigator to turn up information about your previous employment or your private life that could be used against you. In addition, some alleged harassers take the offensive, filing defamation cases against the target who accuses them of sexual harassment. Although they usually lose, these cases are expensive to defend both emotionally and monetarily. See Appendix for a chart of legal remedies against sexual harassment.

Prevention of Further Harassment

In order to set up a work situation free from harassment, employers or schools are *required* to take specific steps:

1. Publicize the laws forbidding harassment at work and school.
2. Train supervisors and other staff to increase their awareness of what constitutes harassment.
3. Set up grievance procedures so that anyone being harassed can make a complaint within the organization.

If You Think You've Harassed Someone

If you think someone might have felt harassed by something you did, you should ask the person privately, "It occurred to me that last week when I . . . (describe what you did), it might have made you uncomfortable. Did that bother you?" If the other person says no, you might want to double-check and say, "Are you sure?" If the person says yes, you can consider apologizing. You might add, "Please tell me if anything I do offends you. I'd rather know so I can change."

Be aware that if you are found guilty of sexual harassment you can be charged with a crime.

Unethical "Helping" Professionals

There is a kind of sexual harassment that violates the codes of ethics in the helping professions. In all but the rarest of cases, this harassment leaves the victim even more wounded than when she sought help. Its perpetrators, who are therapists, clergymen, physicians, and other professionals, make sexual advances toward patients or clients to such an extent that hundreds are still trying to recover from the damage. While men are occasionally abused in this way, again the victims are overwhelmingly female. This kind of exploitation is so common that ethics committees in the helping professions are busily updating their ethics guidelines.

Peter Rutter, M.D., exposes the extent of this epidemic in his book *Sex in the Forbidden Zone*. Rutter talks about the confusion of sex with power in our society and the sexual sickness that encourages this attitude in all of us. Many women think at first that their situation is different ("My therapist is not abusive, he loves me.") But after interviewing hundreds of victims from all walks of life, Rutter defines sex in the forbidden zone:

> *Sexual behavior between a man and a woman who have a professional relationship based on trust, specifically when the man is the woman's doctor, psychotherapist, pastor, lawyer, teacher, or workplace mentor.*[21]

Once again the dysfunctional attitudes of society encourage both the professional *and* the victim to become involved when sexual feelings arise. The whole culture encourages men to challenge women's intimate boundaries. Rutter believes that our society discourages men from learning to empathize with women. He laments this loss for men as well, because " . . . they have so much more to offer women than predatory sexual opportunism."

But society also programs women to respond positively to men in power, to feel tremendously flattered by the advances of a male professional. Many women, pondering the months and years required for them to recover from this exploitation, say they were almost in a trance at the time. Even if the man physically repelled them, some felt they could do nothing but go along. Some even recognized that they were initiating a sexual relationship in order to repeat seductive patterns of their childhood.

We hold adults responsible for sexually exploiting children; we have to hold professionals responsible for exploiting vulnerable adults, for not maintaining their professional ethics. In the overwhelming majority of cases, survivors claim that the experience reaped bitter consequences ranging from the inability to complete psychotherapy to the failure to obtain an adequate divorce settlement because of retaliation from attorneys who were their former lovers. They frequently mourn the fact that they have been unable to form another relationship for years afterward without seeking out the role of victim.

In the most common professional exploitation, seduction—not force—is involved. The question the woman needs to ask is not, "What can I *say* to respond to such a dilemma?" The issue is, "How can I get hold of my *feelings* in order to see clearly that I am dealing with an exploiter?" What should you do if you're faced with professional abuse?

Mental Health Professionals

Cassie, a woman twenty years old, has been consulting a psychologist for several years. He's never seduced her. In fact, he merely kisses her on the cheek when she arrives and when she leaves, and asks her about her sex life. (In his words, "Who have you "f___ed" lately?) She did not think that this behavior was a big deal, but she was not getting better. A friend urged her to find another therapist, but she said her parents liked the psychologist and wouldn't pay for anyone else.

I asked a reputable psychiatrist what he thought a patient should say if a therapist suggested anything sexual. He replied, "Good-bye." Noted sexologist William Masters believes that any professional who becomes sexually involved with a patient should not only be pursued and sued for malpractice, but also should be prosecuted for statutory rape.[22] Many professionals agree. If a mental health professional gives you any sexual attention, whether it makes you uncomfortable or not, it is a serious violation of that person's professional ethics. Some mentally ill women have remained untreated for years because a lack of trust resulted from this kind of abuse. In the depression that may follow the sudden realization that they have been used, a number of women commit suicide.

There is no excuse, there is no possible reason for such sexual attention. All the rationalizations a therapist may offer are completely self-serving. A therapist says this is part of treatment? If sex is so therapeutic, why doesn't he offer this kind of therapy to everyone regardless of age or sexual attractiveness? He is exploiting his client, who should leave at once and call one of the resources in the Appendix to find a new therapist. Emotional support is available from local crisis hotlines, counseling centers, or women's groups, who can offer perspective (male victims should try these numbers for a referral). Local professional associations can help determine where to file a complaint. A therapist's title or status is no reason for awe—he is no more than an abuser with a degree.

Physicians, Nurses, Dentists, and Other Medical Professionals

It is unethical for any person who is treating you medically to give you sexual attention of any kind. Such attention can put you in the difficult position that, if either of you changes your mind, you may be rejected and, in retaliation, denied competent medical care. All sorts of possibilities arise when you mix sex with a professional relationship. However attractive your physician might be, however strong your need for fantasy and love, you're taking a big chance if you willingly becoming involved. Such liaisons almost never develop into healthy and lasting relationships, and it is almost always the one without power who does the suffering.

The sexual harasser sometimes knows just how far to go for gratification without getting into trouble. In the case of Jody, for example, her dentist brushed up against her breasts on three occasions. Not knowing what to do, she just changed dentists. But for years she questioned herself—had she been accurate? Was it just an accident? Or had she done something to encourage him? Every time she thought about the experience, she felt so ashamed and embarrassed that she told no one until years later.

It is the ultimate cruelty for anyone you're depending upon to proposition you sexually during the stress of a crisis. Some exploiters have waited until a patient was desperate or even suicidal before making a seductive move. If you are in a situation in which you can immediately get help elsewhere, this would be the wisest course of action. The seducer knows what he is doing. He is like a predatory animal lurking near wounded prey: he knows you are vulnerable.

Attorneys

Any professional relationship is better off uncontaminated by extra kinds of emotional baggage. What if you have an affair with your attorney and your relationship sours before you go to court? What if the attorney thinks his first bill was unduly low and revises it upward? If you argue, will he begin to identify with your estranged spouse's cause? As needy as human beings can be, they should watch out for any situations that mix personal with professional roles. You may be able to handle such mixing, but if the other person cannot, trouble could result.

Treatment for Sexual Harassers

Some harassers may be helped by counseling. There are two types available: Educational counseling to teach the harasser appropriate behaviors, and psychotherapy through a mental health professional, to get at the underlying needs that lead to exploitation of other people. Compulsive harassers may be sexual addicts. (See Appendix for resources.)

Assertiveness on Tap

The assertive attitude does not always have to be put into words, but it can be there for you to draw upon. If you are aware of your rights and you think you're worth it, even your body language tends to convey your intention to stay within your role as a student, employee, parishioner, or client. Some potential harassers will notice, and it will be more difficult for a potential abuser to fantasize about your being passively cooperative.

Construct a Conversation to Confront the Harasser

You are a student at State University, planning a career in medicine and thinking you're finally on your way. Your professor, Dr. Ronald, teaches the most important chemistry courses at State U. One day you are working late in the lab and he comes in, puts his arm around you, and under the guise of trying to "help" you, rubs your inner thigh. You get up to get some chemicals off the shelf. The first time you think this must have been an accident, but later he repeats this behavior, until one day when you're standing in his office he reaches over and starts playing with the zipper of your jeans. You back up and, fearful of flunking chemistry, make an excuse to leave. You hope it's all over, and try to go to the lab with someone else whenever possible, but your schedule requires you to be there alone sometimes. Your worst fears develop when, one evening, Dr. Ronald comes up behind you unexpectedly and puts his hand on your cheek, turning your face up, bends over, and kisses you. Alarm shoots through your body. You make an excuse to leave. Your college plans seem to be dissolving into a disaster you can't escape. You contact a sexual harassment adviser on the campus, who explains several options to you. You decide to confront Dr. Ronald. Using the three levels of confrontation on page 125, write in a conversational tone what you could say to Dr. Ronald.

1. Describe what happened: Dr. Ronald, . . .

2. Describe how you feel and the effect this has had on you:

3. Describe what you would like to happen:

Notes

1. Barbara A. Gutek, *Sex and the Workplace* (San Francisco: Jossey-Bass Publishers, 1985), 58.

2. A. L. Culbertson, P. Rosenfeld, S. Booth-Kewley, and P. Magnusson, "Assessment of Sexual Harassment in the Navy: Result of the 1989 Navy-wide survey. (TR92-11) San Diego: Naval Personnel Research and Development Center, 1992, as quoted in Louise F. Fitzgerald, "Sexual Harassment: Violence Against Women in the Workplace," *American Psychologist* 48, no. 10 (1993); 1070; Susan Strauss, *Sexual Harassment and Teens: A Program for Positive Change* (Minneapolis: Free Spirit Publishing Company, 1992), 11.

3. Susan L. Webb, *Step Forward: Sexual Harassment in the Workplace, What You Need to Know*, (Mastermedia Limited, 1991) p. xviii. n.p.

4. Strauss, *Sexual Harassment and Teens: A Program for Positive Change*, 15.

5. United States Merit Systems Protection Board, 1981, 1987. U.S. Merit Systems Protection Board (1987) Sexual harassment of federal workers: An update. Washington, D.C.: U.S. Government Printing Office.

6. Ronni Sandross, "Sexual Harassment in the Fortune 500," *Working Woman* 13 (December 1988), 69.

7. Webb, *Step Forward*; Fitzgerald, "Sexual Harassment: Violence Against Women in the Workplace," 1070–1076.

8. Gutek, *Sex in the Workplace*, 56–57.

9. Billie W. Dziech and Linda Weiner, *The Lecherous Professor: Sexual Harassment on Campus* (Boston: Beacon Press, 1984); Gutek, *Sex in the Workplace*.

10. Richard Barickman et al., "An Ecological Perspective to Understanding Sexual Harassment," in Michele A. Paludi, ed., *Ivory Power: Sexual Harassment on Campus* (Albany, N.Y.: State University of New York Press, 1990), xi–xix.

11. Mary Koss, "Changed Lives: The Psychological Impact of Sexaual Harassment," in Paludi, ed., *Ivory Power*, 73–92.

12. Attorney Lois Vander Waerdt of the Employment Partnership, personal communication, January 23, 1995.

13. Antonia Abbey, "Sex Differences in Attributions for Friendly Behavior: Do Males Misperceive Females' Friendliness?" *Journal of Personality and Social Psychology* 42, no. 5 (May 1982): 830.

14. Vita C. Rabionwitz, "Coping with Sexual Harassment," in Paludi, ed., *Ivory Power*, 113.

15. Dziech and Weiner, *Lecherous Professor*, 75–76.

16. Judith Martin, *Miss Manners' Guide for the Turn-of-the Millennium* (New York: Pharos Books, 1989) 212.

17. Elissa Clarke, *Stopping Sexual Harassment: a Handbook* (Detroit: Labor and Education Research Project, 1981), 12.

18. Personal correspondence with Lois Vander Waerdt, President, The Employment Partnership, January 15, 1995.

19. Mary Rowe, "Dealing With Sexual Harassment," *Harvard Business Review* 59, no. 3 (May–June 1981), 42.

20. Lois Vander Waerdt, The Employment Partnership.

21. Peter Rutter, *Sex in the Forbidden Zone* (Los Angeles: Jeremy P. Tarcher, 1989), 22–23.

22. William Masters, as quoted in *Contemporary Sexuality* 25, no. 6 (June 1991), 2.

7

Avoiding
Acquaintance Rape

it will do us large to recall
when the animal in us rises
that all women are someone's
mother, sister, wife, or daughter
and are not fruit to be stolen when hungry.[1]
—HAKI R. MADHUBUTI

What are the odds of a woman or man being raped in the United States? Averaging the findings of several recent surveys, experts judge that the chances of an American woman being raped in her lifetime are one in four. The odds are about one in three that she will be the target of either an actual or an *attempted* rape. The rate of rape in the United States is estimated to be more than 20 times that of Japan and 13 times that of Britain.[2] The National Crime Victimization Survey, long criticized by rape experts for underreporting rape, estimates that there is a rape every 3.5 minutes in the United States.[3] Surprisingly, the FBI estimates that around ten percent of all sexual assaults are against men.[4] Imagine hearing an alarm go off every 3.5 minutes, no matter where you are, when one of your fellow citizens is being sexually penetrated by force.

Legal definitions of rape vary from state to state. In most states, the charge of rape centers around penile-vaginal penetration. This definition is influenced by our notions that nothing else is "real" sex and causes a problem for men who have been raped or women who have been sexually assaulted in other ways. Sexual intercourse is considered rape in most states if the victim was:

- Fearful for her/his life or safety
- Coerced, with words, threats, physical restraint, physical violence, with or without use of a weapon

- Unable to consent, such as being asleep, incapacitated, or physically helpless due to drugs/alcohol
- Younger than that state's age of consent
- Mentally incompetent

Sexual assault has many variations, such as forced oral or anal penetration and vaginal penetration with objects. Assault also takes place when the rapist urges chemical substances on the victim, rendering the victim unable to resist, or when the victim submits under verbal threat of physical harm. Until the late eighties, in most states it was legal for a man to force sex upon his wife. Marital rape is now a crime in all 50 states.[5]

Rape-Free Societies

Although you may not believe the facts that are corroborated from years of study by scores of experts, the truth is that rape is not a part of human nature; it is an act found largely in violent cultures. In fact, there are societies, such as the Ashanti of West Africa and the Mbuti Pygmies, in which rape is either absent or rare. Anthropologist Peggy Sanday studied over 156 societies. In rape-free cultures she found that women participate in religion, politics, or economics as freely as men do. Relationships among the people in low-rape societies are nonviolent, and women are respected throughout.[6]

The Culture of Rape

Once your consciousness is raised about the way our society encourages rape, you may feel yourself to be a misfit. In a way, you are. One of the symptoms of a rape-prone society is that, when someone becomes alarmed about it, she is often treated like a far-out, overly sensitive person who is making a mountain out of a molehill. Rape-prone attitudes are so ingrained that even nonviolent Americans have distorted opinions on the subject. And the experts believe that trying to change individuals will not solve the problem unless the social and cultural institutions that support rape are transformed.[7]

Rape can be committed against any person, regardless of age, income, gender, or ethnic group. It is always extremely disruptive to the emotions and can cause serious psychological aftereffects in both female and male victims. Virtually all male rape victims are penetrated anally or orally by men; in a very few cases men are raped by women. It is possible for males to become sexually aroused without wanting to have intercourse; in rare instances, a man has been tied down and tortured, sometimes for hours, while one or more women had intercourse with him. Some of these men have required extensive sex therapy to overcome the dysfunctions that resulted from these experiences. It helps men to feel empathy with rape victims if they realize that rape is a violation that can happen to anyone.

The rape of one woman causes all men to be suspect. A woman's fear injures innocent men because she will question their motives. In addition to the fact that males can be rape victims, they suffer from living in a society where half the population has reason to be resentful, suspicious, and scared. People who have not been through the experience often do not understand the rape victim's feelings. The emotions associated with being physically violated are difficult to comprehend, particularly when a person has been socialized to think that "getting a piece" is always hilarious good fun. After all, doesn't everyone want to "rip off a little"? Here is a rape survivor's description of how she felt a month after a date raped her and forced her to have oral sex:

> *I cut off all my hair. I did not want be attractive to men. I started wearing real androgynous clothes—nothing tight, nothing revealing—and reduced my makeup to almost nil. I just wanted to look neutered for a while because that felt safer.*[8]

This woman did not date again for several years. Both men and women survivors of rape report a variety of intense reactions, most of which involve fear and loss of self-esteem. They often need counseling to help them adjust.

Again, remember that the need for rape-prevention skills does not in any way suggest that the victim is to blame. We need not blame people for being assaulted to show that they might learn to reduce their chances that assault will happen to them.

Victims and Survivors

Workers in the field of sexuality prefer to use the term *survivor* in place of *victim* whenever possible. The word *survivor* emphasizes prevailing over the experience. When I am discussing ways to avoid being victimized, I may use the word *victim*. But *survivor* is a word that can make a profound difference when applied to oneself. I recall a quotation from some unnamed source: "Life is the transcendence of loss." I would rephrase it to say that *successful* life is the transcendence of loss. The person who is victimized loses a feeling of safety in this world. Some of that loss can be reclaimed. But all of life involves losing and overcoming—losing friends, losing a love relationship, losing a chance or an opportunity. We can overcome loss and become survivors.

How the Media Influence the Rape Culture

We are socialized to believe that men scare women, but not the reverse. This training is the reason unusual movies with violent *women* scaring *men*, like *Fatal*

Attraction and *The Last Seduction* are so frightening—they contradict the script that Hollywood has used for fifty years to earn so many millions of our dollars.

I cannot remember when, as a child, I first saw a film about a scared, helpless woman trying to escape from a horrible crazy man who might do—who knows what?—to her. Even Dracula stalked terrified, screaming women to commit the clearly Freudian deed of sinking his teeth into their necks while they moaned in—ecstasy? I could not fathom the fact that the bad man scaring the poor, weak woman was merely an attitude of fiction. This terrified woman with a bad man seemed like reality to me. Of course, learns the child in America, women are scared and men are the bad guys.

Today such plots are far more frequent. Notice the pictures of brutal, vicious men and helpless women on the fronts of VCR tapes in your video store. The sexual script is clear: It's exciting to see men chase helpless women, especially with sex on their minds. Children don't know that's only fiction—they decide that's how life is. They absorb the myths of how men and women are supposed to act.

Media dramas and novels subtly weave rape into plots; often they actually romanticize it. Even in the early seventies, force was used in about one-third of the sex scenes in hard-core paperback books, almost always by a male to coerce a female into sex against her will.[9] Recent storylines employ force much more often, and blatant pictures of coercion are common even on magazine covers. Bondage and domination increased between 1970 and 1981 to 17.2 percent of the magazine covers of heterosexual pornographic magazines.[10] Such statistics about pornography may not be surprising, but inside the covers of mainstream novels, scenes of rape and near-rape also abound. A typical "love" scene occurs in Hilary Norman's novel, *In Love and Friendship*, in which a rape makes an estranged marriage more spicy:

> *He laughed harshly. He yanked at her skirt, and she heard the fabric ripping and felt small pain as his fingers tore roughly at her panties. His hands moved to her shoulders, pushing them down so violently that her head banged against the floor, and he kneed her legs apart. Suddenly, all the fight seemed to go out of her. She stared into his face in disbelief. "Don't do this, Andreas. I'm begging you." Her voice sounded flat. "If you rape me," she said, "how will I ever forgive you?"*[11]

But of course, she does, and very romantically so. When she forgives him, the reader is not surprised; that's our national script. Countless novels and soaps contain romantic rapes where the woman forgives the rapist, thereby reinforcing the all-American theme that women really like it rough.

Even Scarlett O'Hara was raped by Rhett Butler in perhaps our best-known film, *Gone With the Wind*. And she loved it, which further confuses viewers. Watching *Dangerous Liaisons* or *Doctor Zhivago*, few moviegoers realized that in each film, a young teenager was raped. But soon after the sexual coercion, each girl began to like sex and wait for the man's secret visits. Viewers forgot that they had seen a rape, so seductively did these young maidens smile over their new-found sexuality.

This portrayal of females loving sexual force is one of the most dangerous ways to depict rape. In *War of the Roses*, a husband attempts to rape his wife and she fights fiercely, then suddenly stops fighting and loves it. *The Last Seduction* contained a long scene in which a woman was bent over on a desk with her buttocks bared, screaming, "Rape me! Rape me!" and the man complied. Except, of course, because she asked for it, that was not rape, further confusing the viewer. Research shows that when women are portrayed as liking rape, it changes the attitudes of even nonviolent men to the point that they aren't as shocked by rape and more often think women like it.[12]

Then there are the humorous rapes. You've no doubt forgotten them because they are comedies. For example, in *Robin Hood, Prince of Thieves* there is a prolonged rape attempt by the Sheriff in which Maid Marian keeps her legs together. When her legs finally part, there is a loud laugh track. Of course, she's rescued—by a man. Message: Rape is funny, and women are so helpless that they cannot defend themselves against a violent man without a male protector.

In a rape-prone culture like ours, it's easy for these things to go right over our heads. Nobody is going to chat socially about her rape, and certainly no man is going to confide that he has been overpowered by another man. Rape is an intrusion into the most private part of the self—too personal to mention to any but the most trusted others. Rape survivors, like people who have been infected with STDs, rarely feel comfortable talking about it. Your society propagandizes you to view rape as a rare attack by a crazed stranger. But it has happened to someone on your street, in your class, or at your work.

How Can Rape Be So Common?

Few Americans can truly integrate the fact that rape happens to one of four American women. In an extensive, well-controlled study of over 6,000 college students, Mary Koss came up with the finding that 25 percent of college women have either suffered rape or attempted rape *between the ages of fourteen and twenty-one*.[13] Fifteen percent of the sample were actually raped, and this within a period of a few years.

The high rape rate among certain athletes is cited over and over:

> *Football and basketball players representing NCAA-affiliated schools were reported to police for sexual assault approximately 38% more often than the average male on a college campus, as measured by an FBI survey.*[14]

One in twelve men in Koss's survey admitted to acts that meet legal definitions of rape. Remember, this was a far-reaching and comprehensive survey sampling students from a variety of schools in all sections of the United States. The reason the mind rejects these findings, which occur over and over in other studies, is that we think of rapists as sex-crazed madmen who spring from the darkness onto strangers.

But most rape is committed by someone known to the victim. Nearly all teenage victims know their attackers. By far the majority of reported rapes on college campuses are committed by fraternity members. There is even an entire book entitled *Fraternity Gang Rape*[15] The author cited more than seventy-five documented cases of gang rape on college campuses by June 1988, when a few schools began to become concerned and take complaints seriously.[16]

During one recent year, two midwestern universities reported serious acquaintance rape problems—typical of large universities. On one campus 400 acquaintance rapes had been reported during the year; 75 percent were committed by fraternity men on that campus.[17] The other university reported that one of every six of its women students had been sexually assaulted during their brief stay at the university, and fraternity members were involved in three-fifths of these assaults.[18] These statistics are reflected in crime data from numerous other campuses. A fraternity house is one of the few places in this country where admiration of alcohol and sexual prowess combine with permission to engage in impulsive behaviors in a basically unsupervised environment. Hopefully, the efforts of fraternities to improve these conditions will have an impact on the safety of college women.

It can't be so, some say. Surely this rape publicity is a plot by a group of man-hating women who don't shave their legs and who burn their bras. Where did these universities obtain such findings? The answer is relatively simple: Most people do not report rape. Only 5 percent of rape victims are believed to report the incident to the police. And most Americans do not realize that all forced sex is rape. The Koss study found that *only 27 per cent of the women raped identified themselves as rape victims.* They often suffered from fear, anger, and other possible aftereffects of rape, but they were as confused as the rest of society about the definition of rape. They usually blamed themselves for what happened. When counselors encouraged some of the survivors to label their experience as an actual rape, they usually felt better. How does rape by an acquaintance actually happen? Here's Wendy's story:

> *I used to go out with this guy for a while, and then we stopped seeing each other. I was not that serious. Then one day there was a knock at my door, and it was him. He said he just wanted to talk. I didn't think anything; I let him in. He started kissing me. I told him to stop. I pushed him away. He kept on. He said, "You know you love it." I said, "No, I don't. Stop it!" But he kept on. He pushed me down on the bed. I kept trying, but I couldn't . . . I couldn't get him to stop. He . . . raped me. All the time he kept telling me how much I wanted it. He even saw me the next day*

and he said, "That wasn't rape." And I said, "Oh, yes it was." But he didn't even listen to me, he had made up his mind. He thought I loved it. I . . . haven't gone out with anyone since. I stay home a lot.

Rape Attitude Checklist

Acquaintance rapists *seem* to be regular guys. Their beliefs at first glance don't seem rape-prone. What are your beliefs about rape? Answer true or false:

1. __ Rape is a part of male nature going back to the cavemen.

2. __ The overwhelming majority of rapes are committed by a male stranger against a female.

3. __ All women like a man who is pushy and forceful.

4. __ A promiscuous person cannot be raped.

5. __ A man cannot be raped.

6. __ If a woman fights, a man cannot penetrate her.

7. __ A woman often causes her own rape by retreating from an agreement to have sex.

8. __ Most women have a secret desire to be raped.

9. __ Women say no when they mean yes.

10. __ It's up to a woman to keep things under control.

11. __ If a couple have ever had consensual sex before, forced intercourse between them later is not rape.

12. __ A woman often causes her own rape by going into an unsafe situation such as a bad neighborhood or bar.

13. __ A woman who leads a man on shouldn't be surprised if she gets what she deserves.

14. __ The way women dress, they are just asking to be raped.

15. __ Men are just naturally going to try to get women drunk to see how much sex they can get.

16. __ A "real" man pushes when the partner says no.

17. __ Rapists are crazed by sexual desire.

18. __ Women who drink too much deserve what they get.

19. __ There is a fine line between seduction and rape, and a man can't always be expected to know where one ends and the other begins.

20. __ There may be male rape victims, but they are either gay or weak.

Did you mark any of the above as true? All of these statements are *myths* about rape, but they are common beliefs in our country. Rape is no more a part of male nature than killing babies is a part of female nature. While some men and women fantasize about being raped, fantasies are under their control; no one actually *desires* to be raped—which represents a total *lack* of control. Rape survivors said no and meant it, and the acquaintance rapist often did not believe them. Women who mean no certainly attempt to communicate that message to the rapist, but he either doesn't care or doesn't interpret her refusal as a true rejection.

Such is our victim-blaming mentality that, if a rapist did not leap out of the darkness, it must be the woman's fault. After all, she used to date him, or she shouldn't have stayed behind at the party, or she shouldn't have had those two drinks or worn that sweater. But if she knew him and particularly if she's been kissing and petting with him, then if he forces her . . . that isn't rape, is it? Yes, it is. If she says no and tries to stop him, it is rape. "Ever since Adam took his first bite of the apple," say rape experts Kathryn Quina and Nancy Carlson, "women have been accused of causing otherwise normal men to lose control."[19] Society and even the criminal justice system often blame women for causing their own rape by entering vulnerable situations. Yes, hitchhikers and women who go into other dangerous situations may be raped. But just being ignorant or naive is not a rapable offense. Many women are raped trying to get to or from work. Rape happens in suburban as well as urban areas, and not always in a place thought to be dangerous.

Studies of men who have committed rape show that they believe most of the above myths and think it is normal for sex and aggression to be mixed up together. There have been several surveys of men who rate themselves "likely to rape" if they could get by with it.[20] Repeatedly these men have said they believe the rape myths and they show a callous attitude toward rape. Many men also misread women's signals consistently, and there is plenty of research to back up this fact.[21] If she squeezes his hand in the movie, doesn't she want what he wants? This kind of misunderstanding is very frequent in male-female relationships today.

Michael S. Kimmel, one of the nation's foremost educators on men and masculinity, doesn't pull any punches when describing prorape attitudes:

> *Women's sense of entitlement to desire is drowned out by the incessant humming of male desire, propelling him ever forward. . . . One fraternity at a college I was lecturing at last year offered seminars to pledges on dating etiquette that appropriated the book of business advice called* Getting to Yes. *Sometimes that hum can be so loud that it drowns out the actual voice of the real live woman he's with. Men suffer from socialized deafness, a hearing impairment that strikes only when women say "no."*[22]

In pure self-defense, women need to become aware of what men see as seductive, regardless of whether they intend it to be. If society does not make changes fast enough to make a safe environment for you, you will increase your odds of being safe by making some accommodations.

The rapist may be morally and psychologically abnormal, but statistically he is not. That is, rape-prone attitudes are so common in our society that they may be the norm. Scientist Neil Malamuth reported that 35 percent of the college men he interviewed said they would force sex on a woman if they were guaranteed they could get away with it.[23] Similar results show up in surveys of teenage and adult males throughout our society.

After all, is recovering from rape such a big deal? Just talk to a man who loves a rape survivor, whose beloved may have so much difficulty trusting him that their relationship cannot grow. Talk to survivors who have needed counseling, who have been afraid to go out, and who have not been able to trust men. A country that tells all its men to score with women cannot be expected to believe that its women really don't feel the same. Aren't the victims just scoring, too? One study of college males found 83 percent agreeing to the following statement: "Some women look like they're just asking to be raped."[24] Although certain clothing styles may seem seductive, don't forget: In some societies, women can walk around bare from the waist up and not get raped. The idea that anyone is asking to be raped because of her clothes is completely ludicrous; that she wants consenting sex may not even be accurate. Where respect for individual rights is strong, rape does not occur regardless of what women wear.

A sexually frustrated male can hardly be expected to control himself, can he? That's another one of the myths. Rape is not primarily a sexual act. Most stranger rapists have sexual access to girlfriends or wives. Rape is primarily a crime of violence. Ask any incarcerated rapist and he will tell you that anger and power, not lust, were his reasons.

The suggestions in this chapter apply largely to rape by someone known to the victim—*acquaintance* rape. While sexual assertiveness is possible against stranger rapists, it obviously has more potential for helping prevent acquaintance rape. Most acquaintance rapes happen in the rapist's territory—his apartment, for example. The time has come to treat a stranger who wants to date you as an unknown quantity. Yet we are socialized to trust people we date. And a major problem is simply our definition of knowing someone. You can be acquainted with someone whom you do not know well enough to be alone with him.

How to Recognize a Potential Rapist

Robin Warshaw, author of *I Never Called it Rape*, offers convincing advice on how to avoid acquaintance rape, based on the experience of rape counselors and rape survivors.[25] She suggests that you learn to recognize the behaviors common to the potential rapist. Do not be surprised if you've seen these behaviors fairly often. Research clearly shows them to be present in rape- and abuse-prone personalities. Warshaw advises that you run, not walk, from any man who displays any of these characteristics:

1. *Emotionally abuses you** through insults, belittling comments, ignoring your opinion, or by acting sulky or angry when you initiate an action or idea.
2. *Tells you who you may be friends with, how you should dress, or tries to control* other elements of your life or relationship. He insists on picking the movie you'll see, the restaurant where you'll eat, and so on.
3. *Talks negatively about women* in general.
4. *Gets jealous* when there's no reason.
5. *Drinks heavily or uses drugs* and tries to get you intoxicated.
6. *Berates you* for not wanting to get drunk, get high, have sex, or go with him to an isolated personal place such as his room, your apartment, or the like.
7. *Refuses to let you share* any of the expenses of a date and gets angry if you offer to pay.
8. *Is physically violent* to you or others, even if it's "just" grabbing and pushing to get his way.
9. *Acts in an intimidating way* toward you: sits too close, uses his body to block your way, speaks as if he knows you much better than he does, touches you when you tell him not to.
10. *Is unable to handle sexual and emotional frustrations* without becoming angry.
11. *Doesn't view you as an equal,* either because he's older or because he sees himself as smarter or socially superior.
12. *Has a fascination with weapons.*
13. *Enjoys being cruel* to animals, children, or people he can bully.

If you find that you repeatedly become involved with men who have any of these characteristics, you must consider why you *choose* this kind of person. After a few times, it is not just chance. You would not choose to be raped, and you need to look at why you're choosing abusive men. A person with self-esteem does not stick around to be demeaned and frightened. Find yourself a good support group, or go to a therapist or counselor to help you understand this self-destructive behavior. You may want to read some books about addictive relationships. One example is *Men Who Hate Women and the Women Who Love Them.*[26]

Talking to Rape-Prone Males

It is far better to ignore and steer clear of such men as Warshaw describes above. The major distortion in the minds of most acquaintance rapists is their tendency to interpret friendliness as seduction. She may be refusing him, but she won't be able

---

* Italics are mine

to get her resistance across because he's not reading the message she's sending. This misunderstanding of a woman's intentions is even present in many nonrapists, because the entire culture encourages it. Look for Warshaw's clues early and get yourself out of the situation. Don't be challenged by wanting to shape this guy up with your assertiveness. *He does not perceive reality the way you do.* Don't hold on to the hope that, because he's so good-looking or so popular, you can bring out his decent inner nature if you're just nice to him. When you act nice toward him, especially if you've tolerated *any* put-downs such as outlined above, he may mistakenly read this as a signal that you are fair game for more. However, you may find you are in a situation you feel you cannot leave. If you want to establish yourself as unavailable, then assertive responses may be able to help you get that across.

When Someone Tries to Get You Drunk

Let's say that you attend a party at a friend's house, and a nice-looking guy keeps making eye contact with you. At first you are interested. But after listening to him awhile, you note that he drops a few remarks about stupid women and is trying to get you to drink more than you want. You've tried walking to the other side of the room, but he follows you. He begins to engage the other people in your group in conversation about you:

He: This little gal here, she's just a party pooper, she won't take any of this good stuff (pushes a bottle at you and grins).

You: I don't want any. (You turn and walk away.)

Never smile at the joke. He may be one of the millions who misinterpret a smile as a come-on. You're not pleased—you must be totally clear.

When Someone Gets Too Close Physically

What if someone in a restaurant booth keeps getting closer to you than you want? Some men are sensitive to mild assertion such as your continually scooting away. The next level of assertiveness is to say, "Please stop sitting so close."

If that doesn't stop him, rape counselors advise that you escalate: Leave, push him away, or tell him, "Get off!" He's already showing insensitivity to your rights. A considerate man who wants to impress you starts with conversation, not with physically pushing you. If you've been dreaming of a great relationship, this can never be one.

Suppose a man in whom you are not interested continually puts his arm around your waist, or comes too close, or keeps putting his hand on your thigh, although you move away and otherwise resist. Rape prevention experts recommend that you speak sharply: "Stop that!" If he does not stop, they advise you to escalate: "Stop that! Take your hands off me!"

That's not nice, and that's not sweet—why, that sounds like some kind of far-out women's libber, no doubt. If you repel this intruder, someone might say you weren't even *polite*. Or someone might not even *like* you. Or even call you a *bitch*, heaven forbid! Keep your priorities straight. The experts advise: *better rude than raped*. If you are uncomfortable defending your sexual boundaries, it is not that this advice is too strong. It's that you are quite naturally brainwashed to believe you shouldn't assert yourself. You've bought the cultural myths about assertive women being aggressive. *The highest rates of acquaintance rape occur to inexperienced and naive young women who were trying to be nice.* Any rape education expert at a college will tell you that the biggest challenge in working with women is helping them to feel comfortable taking their own power. Good men who are caring and respectful will not judge you in the least for repelling such a person. "There is no downside to owning your own strength; the only people who don't like it are abusers."[27]

It is not unfeminine to have self-esteem. It is feminine to defend yourself. It is feminine to have courage. Your pioneer or native American ancestors, your slave ancestors, or your immigrant ancestors were strong women. Feel them there with you inside your mind. You need to be furious with anyone who violates your boundaries. You need to feel, "How dare you!"

When a Date Is Excessively Jealous

How can you answer a date who shows excessive jealousy? Be very alert to any kinds of jealous remarks, such as "Why the hell are you talking to *him*, when you came with *me*?" Don't start defending yourself. There's no point in trying to reassure a person with such distorted attitudes. If your date talks like this, don't even risk going home with him. Try to get a ride with someone you trust. It is not normal to restrict a date from even talking to another person. That's the red flag of an abuser waving in your face.

These are not relationships you should work to improve, but nonrelationships, and you want to make that crystal clear. These men are showing signs of being abusers and may be more dangerous than an obscene phone caller or an exhibitionist. Don't smile, don't engage in polite conversation as if the man had not said or done something on Warshaw's list. You may find yourself confused because these attitudes are so common in men—but so is rape.

When Someone Uses Words or Names that Are Too Familiar

What if someone calls you names you're not comfortable with, or acts as if he knew you better than he does? Get away from him, but not in an isolated spot or alone. If you can't escape quickly, one option is to respond clearly:

"Stop calling me that. I don't like it."

"You don't know me. Leave me alone."

Suppose a man continues to put you down and tries to establish himself as your social superior. This kind of comment is common in acquaintance rapists:

He: (Teasing) You don't know what you're talking about. That's stupid. (He tweaks your hair and grins down at you.)

You: (over your shoulder as you walk away.) I *don't like* to be teased, and I *don't like* to be called names. (No smile.)

Doesn't that sound downright unfriendly? It's not nice to talk tough. But this is a situation that threatens you. It does not call for niceness. You can be nice, too, where it's appropriate. You can still keep "nice" for other times.

The Shock Technique: Call It What It Is

If you are with someone who is trying to force you to have sexual intercourse or oral sex, or keeps acting as if he thinks you want it although you're saying no, some rape prevention trainers suggest you try:

"This is rape! I'm calling the police!"

Remember that these are just options, and one cannot predict what an abuser will do. But considering the kinds of distortions this man has been making, he may need to have it clarified. Another reality jolt that some experts advise is: "Did you know that what you are doing is a felony? You're forcing me and you could go to prison for this!"

Rules for Avoiding Acquaintance Rape

In addition, consider the following suggestions from acquaintance-rape survivors. The advice also applies to gay males, who are raped at an astonishingly high rate in some places:

1. *Set sexual limits and communicate them* to your date. Chapters 4 and 5 show you how to make a policy statement that tells your partner how far you want to go. "I don't want to do more than kiss." If you're kissing but someone goes beyond your limits, say so, even if you have to clear your throat and take a deep breath first: "No. I want to keep my clothes on." If you are really attracted to him and hope to have the relationship grow, you could explain that to him openly: "I hope you understand what I'm trying to say. I really like you a lot, and I hope we keep seeing each other. It's just that I don't want to get sexually involved that far until I know someone really well." Remember, a reasonable person—while he might find those remarks frustrating—will see your rights. He doesn't have to like it, he doesn't even have to date you if instant sex is his requirement. But a reasonable person will not force someone who gives a clear "no" message.

2. *Stay out of isolated spots and do not drive with a stranger* or even with a group that is supposed to meet additional people. In the case histories of acquaintance rape, often a group has disappeared by prearrangement prior to rape. With new dates, drive your car and meet the date somewhere. Insist on going to places that are public, such as out to dinner.

3. *Be definite when you refuse.* Speak firmly and look right at him. Research shows that the more definite the woman's response to his pushing, the more likely it is that the man will believe her.[28]

4. *Notice your fears.* If you're too afraid of displeasing your date, you may not speak assertively. A respectful partner will not treat you badly after you set limits. It is natural for a partner to be frustrated or disappointed—it is *not* natural for him to become angry and demeaning. Don't buy that myth.

5. *Never leave a party or other gathering with a stranger.* Many acquaintance rapes occur when the rapist finds an opportunity to have control over you.

6. *Stay sober.* Safety tests show that alcohol has a negative effect on people long before they think they are drunk. Numerous studies of rape indicate that up to three-fourths of all rapists and victims were using alcohol or other drugs at the time. If you lived in a society where sexual rights were taken for granted, you could feel secure no matter what your chemical condition. You could lie around intoxicated and your date would probably stop if you were able to say no emphatically. But since this is not the case in our society, you're taking a major risk if you use mood-altering chemicals with people of unknown character. Acquaintances who rape often target a female who is drinking. They frequently even plan to ply her with alcohol. Some researchers have found that 75 percent of their sample of college men admitted to using drugs or alcohol to get sex on a date.[29] The idea, as one male student submitted anonymously in my class survey, is "to get a chick wasted and take her home." In one survey of college men, 19 percent said they had given a woman costly drugs so the woman would feel sexually obligated to them, and *10 percent said they had waited in line with other men for their turn to share intercourse with an intoxicated "party girl."*[30] It's important to be drug-free to remain in control of your car, and also to remain in control of your body. It's becoming more and more acceptable to socialize without alcohol or other drugs.

7. *Listen to your vibes.* Trust your gut level feelings about this person. Repeatedly, acquaintance rape survivors say they had a strange feeling about the man, but did not pay any attention to it.

8. *If you're in a new environment, such as college or a foreign country, be especially cautious.* Members of the sorority/fraternity "little sisters" program on college campuses have had one of the highest victimization rates of any group. Several colleges and universities are attempting to cope with this problem; others sweep it under the rug. Foreign media may portray American women as sexually available and cause men to misinterpret your friendliness as seductiveness. After all, if *our films* are shown over there, it is easy to see where they could learn their distortions about Americans.

9. *If you have stopped seeing someone that you really don't like or about whom you don't feel good, don't let him into your place.* A surprising number of acquaintance rapes are committed by an ex-lover or an ex-boyfriend. Stalkers can rape.

10. *Be aware of inequalities in your relationship.* Rape is a violent display of power. Does your partner think his having more money or experience or being older entitles him to power over you?

11. *Be alert to situations that can be misinterpreted.* For example, it might be practical just to sleep on his couch when you're too sleepy to drive home. But the potential rapist may not believe your "no sex" limits—and no one believed her date was a rapist until after it happened. Plan ahead. I especially lament the fact that women must take any responsibility for avoiding victimization by someone else. The responsibility for the rape belongs only to the perpetrator. Once the Knesset in Israel met to discuss the possibility of having a ten o'clock curfew for women, since the rate of rape was increasing. Golda Meir, then the prime minister of Israel, is said to have replied, "The women come home early? They haven't raped anybody. Let the men come home by ten o'clock." But most men have not raped anybody either.

Who Has Successfully Repelled Attempted Rape?

Survivors of stranger and acquaintance rape report that their reaction to the impending assault was fear. Women who have *avoided a rape attempt* have also been studied, to find what successful techniques they may have used and what they felt at the time. Of course, they may have faced drastically different situations than actual rape victims. The use of force by an assailant is still the most important factor determining whether a rape attempt is successful.[31]

Reacting with suspicion and anger instead of fear seems to have made the difference for many of the women who avoided rape. But self-defense trainers complain that it is difficult to get women to act or even *feel* angry about an attack. Women have learned to be nice and simply don't think of fighting back. Imagine yourself yelling, "Get your hands off me!" to an intrusive acquaintance and check to see if you have a fear of coming on too strong. Say it out loud in front of the bathroom mirror when you're alone until you become comfortable with the strength of your voice.

There is no assertive technique that can definitely prevent all *stranger* rape. A person who would sexually assault an unknown person is not usually open to rational persuasion, though a few people have talked a stranger out of attacking them. This does not mean, however, that we know nothing about resisting a rape attempt by an acquaintance. Research with women who have successfully repelled an *acquaintance* rapist indicates that they screamed or ran away more often than did actual rape victims.[32] Talking back to resist a rapist also reduces the chances of rape in some cases.[33] What should you do? Unfortunately, you have to look at all of your options because no one knows the intent of the rapist.

Rape avoiders also felt different *emotions* than did the rape victims. Women who immediately responded to the threat of rape with less fear and more composure were more likely to avoid rape. It could well be that the successful rapists were so intimidating that fear was unavoidable. But feeling strongly about your rights and knowing how to assert yourself will still increase your odds.

Another survey asked avoiders of both stranger and acquaintance rape what strategies they had used.[34] They reported that they used the following more than the victims did:

- Physical and verbal resistance
- More forceful resistance
- More rudeness and hostility prior to attack
- Screaming
- Resisting immediately rather than waiting
- Strong verbal aggression
- Physical fighting
- Running
- The most effective strategy: a combination of physical force and yelling

Although we can learn something from this advice, we must be cautious. Women who raped probably do not have the same options as the women who avoid rape. Studying how people act in traumatic situations is a very complex business. However, recognizing a threatening situation immediately and taking action has usually proved superior to nonresistance. Note also that an intoxicated person probably could not perform the actions that the rape avoiders accomplished.

Beware of Simple Advice

Whereas screaming and yelling may help in many situations, a potential victim needs to think about her effect upon this particular attacker. Physical resistance has stopped some rape attempts, but law enforcement officials warn that oversimplified advice about avoiding rape can be unwise. Research about what *most* rapists do may not apply to *all* individuals. It is asking a lot of a shocked and frightened person to expect her to consider her options calmly. But information can help you to be prepared. Only the potential survivor can decide whether to try one of the options above in these particular circumstances. Just reading this book and evaluating your rape-avoidance strategies will increase your odds of being safe. It's also important to know that, although you cannot control everything that happens to you, you could survive even rape, and you could heal.

How Some Men Justify Rape

Three researchers asked college men what would justify their having intercourse against a woman s wishes.[35] The men rated rape as more justifiable if

- The woman asked the man out
- The man paid for the date rather than splitting it
- They went to his place

Other informal questionnaires show that men may justify rape if:

- She dressed suggestively
- She drank or did drugs

It is appalling that anyone would justify committing a felony over such minor cues. It is outrageous that someone would think you were consenting to sexual intercourse just because you asked him out or because he paid for a date. But over and over, studies indicate that *these confusions exist*. These are the distortions carried around in the heads of thousands of people in your society, and you need to be aware of them. I keep reminding you that what women *intend* and what some men *think* they mean have been repeatedly shown to be quite different. Gay males may also have false expectations, and rape can result.

Making Your Intentions Clear

At the very least, people today need to make their sexual intentions clear when they're in any of the situations above. If your date has been respectful so far, but you don't want to be alone with him yet, you might clarify your intentions as follows:

B: Want to go to my place? I was going to play that tape for you.

A: Not tonight, maybe another time.

B: Why not? It's early.

A: (Looks him straight in the eye.) I'd like to hear the tape, but . . . we don't know each other very well. I'm not sure what it would mean to you if I went to your apartment.

B: (will probably say) I wouldn't think anything!

A: I like you a lot, but I'm not ready to get sexually involved right now. I just thought I'd better say that so we understand each other.

If B is a truthful person, his answer may reassure you. You've made yourself clear. If your date distorts reality the way some acquaintance rapists do, however, he may think you aren't serious.

What do you say if you're not sure what he expects when a man pays for your meals? Thousands of people take others out, enjoy it, and still have clear ideas of everybody's sexual rights in the situation. But you may wonder if your date is one of those men. If you're not sure what he thinks, you could try to clarify:

A: You know, I feel uncomfortable when you keep paying my way. I appreciate you taking me out to such nice places. But I could pay my own way sometimes, too, or treat you.

B: Why? I enjoy it.

A: I know some people think . . . well, it's real important to me to be clear with you. I've met some guys who expect something in return; they misunderstand. I like you a lot, and I want to be clear with you. (Here A may need to make a policy statement. See Chapter 4). I need to know someone well before I decide anything about going to bed with him, do you understand?

A continues to make this policy clear and checks with B on whether he understands. A waits until B says whether he understands. If a person is truthful, he will tell you how he feels and you can make a judgment.

Suppose he really is a great guy and he is shocked that you'd suspect him. He says, "Come on, you surely don't think I'd do anything you did not want to do?" A reasonable person will understand if you explain, in your own words, why you feel you must bring up the subject:

A: It's embarrassing to have to mention things like this, but I think you'll understand. . . . Some of my friends have had things happen when guys misunderstood.

What Men Can Do to Prevent Rape

Preventing rape is not a female responsibility. What will men do to reverse this trend? Some men respect women and contribute nothing but their silence to our rape-prone climate. However, most men can become more sensitive to the factors that encourage a pro-rape atmosphere. Here are some things men can do:

1. *Do not make comments that treat women like objects* and do not brag about sex with them. If someone else does it, a mature and assertive man can disagree:

  "It's not that I'm not listening. I just don't like to hear you talk about her like that."

"That's private, between you and her. I shouldn't be hearing about it."

2. *Do not ply women with drinks* to get them to do things they would not do otherwise. Express your disapproval when other men discuss this behavior:

"You know, guys, I don't go for getting people drunk to get sex. I like my sex to be strictly voluntary."

3. *Do not push women who say no.* Speak up to women who seem to be giving you a double message and ask them which message they really mean:

"You don't sound like you mean it. I need to know what you really want to do."

4. *Do not assume that you and your date want the same amount of sexual intimacy.* Don't assume that her desire for affection means that she wants to have intercourse with you. She may want no sexual contact, or to stop with just kissing. Or, she may want some other kind of sexual contact other than intercourse on which you could mutually agree.

5. *Let your partner know what you want through words,* and don't make her guess:

"I'm not willing to have a relationship without going all the way."
If you feel this way, say so. It may be a selfish viewpoint for a new date, but these words are legal. Or: "I'm willing to wait until you are ready. This is not to say I want to wait, but I will."

6. *Remember that a woman might like you very much and still reject sex with you right now.* She is just expressing her decision not to engage in a particular act at this time. If you push her, you may destroy her affection for you.

7. *Remember that the state of intoxication of you or your partner is not a legal defense for the charge of rape.* Rape is a felony. You can go to prison for doing the very thing that your culture is encouraging you to do: coming on strong and forcefully.

8. *Separate desire from action.* You may not be able to control your desires, but you can control your actions. Sexual excitement does not justify force. Some feminists ask, "If your mother burst in on you while you were getting excited, you could stop, couldn't you?"

9. *Be responsible about the physical advantage you have over most women.* Many survivors of rape report that the fear they felt—based on a man's size and presence—was the reason they did not fight back or struggle. This has sometimes been held up in court in favor of the victim.

10. *Learn to redefine a date in terms of a relationship*: A date can be a success without sex. You'll decrease your chances of getting a disease, and even increase your chances of having a good relationship, if you get to know your date as a person.

11. *Spread the word by talking to other men.* Raping an acquaintance is not only wrong, it's risky for the rapist. DNA testing to prove the identity of a rapist offers hope of far more convictions in the future.

12. *Support organizations of men whose purpose is to reduce violence against women.*

13. *Be a man of honor and tell the truth to a woman you date.* College counselors report that as sexual pressure increases on a date, men may make promises of a loving relationship that they have no intention of keeping.

Writer and publisher Haki Madhubuti makes an impassioned plea for men to view all women as extended family. In "On Becoming Anti-rapist,"[36] his suggestions to African-American men contain deep meanings that speak to all men:

- *Understand that anti-rapist actions are part of the black tradition; being an anti-rapist is in keeping with the best Afrikan culture and with Afrikan family and extended family configurations. Even in times of war we were known to honor and respect the personhood of children and women.*
- *Be bold and strong enough to stop other men (friends and strangers) from raping and to intervene in a rape in process with the fury and destruction of a hurricane against the rapist.*

If You've Been Sexually Abused

People who were sexually abused or assaulted in childhood are more likely to be sexually assaulted than the nonabused.[37] How unfair this seems! If you were abused in childhood, this does not mean you are doomed to have other awful experiences—it means you need to take stock right now of your attitudes. You need to work on feeling *affronted and enraged* if anyone attempts to exploit you sexually. You need to remember that your past might have trained you *not* to get angry over intrusion and coercion—but now you will have to relearn. You also need to take your time before getting sexually involved, because you may have picked up wrong signals about doing what other people want instead of what you want. If you need counseling to understand how you can improve on these matters, check the Appendix for places to go.

If You've Been Raped

Rape does not invariably cause psychological damage. But if you experience any negative changes in your life after a rape, such as depression or excessive fear, even if it seems unrelated to the incident, you may want to check it out with a counselor (see Appendix).

The first thing you need to remember is that your reactions are normal. You may feel numb, scared, depressed, dirty, suspicious, or guilty—or all of those things. That is a stage you will pass through, and you may need help. What happened to you was no accident; someone else made a choice that had nothing to do with you. You may keep going over what you did, trying to make sense of what happened, but there is no sensible reason. Rapists are angry, isolated people who seek to gain control over someone else. The explanation lies in him, not in you. Linda Braswell, in her book, *Quest for Respect*,[38] gently and caringly outlines the steps a rape victim needs to go through in order to become a survivor. She suggests that you first make a list:

- *Whom you can tell*
- *Whom needs to know*
- *Whom you want to know*
- *The right time to tell them*

You should not go through this adjustment by yourself. Consult a rape crisis center if one is available; if not, search for counseling centers, clergy, or other mental health professionals who have special training in dealing with rape survivors.

Braswell explains how you may react at first as you initially blame yourself:

This is the point at which you are likely to seek help. But because the rape is something you are trying hard to forget, you probably don't tell your friends, relatives, or counselors about it, and the help or advice they offer does little good. It takes as much courage to embrace the hurt of the rape as it takes to survive it. It is necessary. It is the only way out of the darkness that has enveloped your life.[39]

Reading Braswell's little book is the next best thing to having a trusted and competent therapist to help you get past the rape. If you are a survivor, I hope you get a copy.

To Avoid Attempted Stranger Rape

It is not the purpose of this book to teach you about physical self-defense. However, there are precautions that will decrease your chances of being raped by a stranger. Answer the checklist on pages 226–228 in the Appendix and see whether you are up to date on measures that you need to build into your lifestyle.

For Help Immediately After a Rape

As much as the rape victim might want to bathe or change clothes or erase all traces of the assault, evidence could be lost in this manner. Anyone who has been raped should seek medical help immediately afterward. It's vital that you see the suggestions in the Appendix. Many communities have access to a rape crisis hotline. Your telephone operator, hospital emergency room, or telephone book should list what is available. If the people you reach do not have a supportive attitude, look elsewhere.

Legal Options

Forcing sexual penetration on another person is a criminal offense. People who have been raped can press criminal and/or civil charges against the person who raped them. Call a rape crisis hotline. (See the Appendix for sources of help.)

Treatment for People Who Use Sexual Force

See the Appendix for sources of treatment for sexual addiction. Referrals might also be obtained from rape crisis hotlines or some of the other resources listed in the Appendix.

Survivors Can Heal

Rape is never in any way the fault of the victim. If rape has happened to you, you can recover from it. I know rape survivors who are now in loving relationships. Even if you did not use any of the above avoidance strategies, if you have been raped and have survived, the offense against you was not your fault. Each circumstance is different and none of us can predict what we would do in a given situation. It is human to react in a confused manner under extreme threat. Even the most well-adjusted people have had many experiences in which they've done something they regretted. I intend the above advice only to help you avoid any further victimization. *Never use it to second-guess what you should have done.* You did the best you could at that time. You are a survivor. Look to the future.

There's one thing that really worries me about some rape survivors. To protect themselves, they block out anything having to do with fear; this denial often results in their taking fewer precautions than a person who has never been raped. I've seen rape survivors get into situations even worse than the one in which they were first victimized. I had a student who was raped at knife-point when she was twelve. At nineteen she was raped again while driving through a dangerous neighborhood at night with her car doors unlocked. I know what was happening: She was so scared that she had to unconsciously block out any thought of being a potential victim. Not facing the fact that someone could enter her car was the only way she could survive psychologically. The fear is so severe in some people that it has to be erased completely. Please, if you have survived rape, make a list of things you need to do, including those in the Appendix, and say them out loud to a dear friend or counselor. Tell the friend you're doing this to help prevent yourself from blocking out safety measures. Focus on how safe you're going to be and mention only positive outcomes. Ask your friend to repeat your precautions back and promise that you'll keep them.

There is hope that we can learn to respect each other's body boundaries and sexual privacy. Not only can you help to defend yourself with assertive techniques, but you can be an instrument of change to protect others.

Powell's Picnic

A man is eating a delicious picnic in his front yard. A well-fed woman suddenly comes up, hits him over the head from behind, and takes his food.

Answer True or False to the following questons:

1. __ He shouldn't have eaten in front of others lest he stimulate their appetites; he should have eaten privately.

2. __ The theft is his fault for flaunting his food.

3. __ The theft is entirely her responsibility.

4. __ Her desire for food is a normal drive, so what can you expect when someone makes food so obvious?

Comments:

Notes

1. Haki R. Madhubuti, "On Becoming Anti-Rapist," in Buchwald, Fletcher, and Roth, eds., *Transforming a Rape Culture*, 169.

2. "Woman under Assault," *Newsweek*, 16 July 1990, 23.

3. Buchwald, Fletcher, and Roth, eds. *Transforming a Rape Culture*, 8.

4. Andrea Parrot, *Acquaintance Rape and Sexual Assault Prevention Manual* (Ithaca, N.Y.: Cornell University, 1990), 8.

5. The National Clearinghouse on Marital and Date Rape in Berkeley, CA, says that there are *some* sex offenses in which the husband is still exempt from prosecution, especially when his wife is mentally or physically, temporarily or permanently, impaired or disabled.

6. Peggy R. Sanday, "The Socio-Cultural Context of a Rape: A Cross-cultural Study," *The Journal of Social Issues* 37 (1981): 5.

7. Lisa A. Goodman et. al., "Male Violence Against Women: Current Research and Future Directions," *American Psychologist* 48, no. 10 (1993): 1055.

8. Warshaw, *I Never Called It Rape*, 33.

9. D. D. Smith, "The Social Content of Pornography," *Journal of Communication* 26 (1976): 16.

10. P. E. Dietz and B. Evans, "Pornographic Imagery and Prevalence of

Paraphilia," *American Journal of Psychiatry* 139 (1982): 1493.

11. Hilary Norman, *In Love and Friendship* (New York: Dell Publishing Company, 1987).

12. N. M. Malamuth and Edward Donnerstein, eds., *Pornography and Sexual Aggression* (New York: Academic Press, 1984).

13. Mary P. Koss, Christine A. Gidycz, and Nadien Wisniewski, "The Scope of Rape: Incidence and Prevalence of Sexual Aggression and Victimization in a National Sample of Higher Education Students," *Journal of Consulting and Clinical Psychology* 55, no. 2 (1987): 162.

14. R. Hoffman, "Rape and the College Athlete: Part One," *Philadelphia Daily News*, 17 March 1986, 104.

15. Peggy R. Sanday, *Fraternity Gang Rape* (New York: New York University Press, 1990).

16. As reported in Sanday's book, *Fraternity Gang Rape*, citing Bernice Sandler's article in the *Atlanta Constitution*, 7 June 1988.

17. " 'Date Rape' Stirring Debate at Mizzou," *St. Louis Post-Dispatch,* 23 April 1989.

18. "Campus Debates Rape Survey Conclusions," *St. Louis Post-Dispatch*, 12 February 1990.

19. Kathryn Quina and Nancy L. Carlson, *Rape, Incest, and Sexual Harassment: A Guide for Helping Survivors* (New York: Praeger, 1989), 35.

20. Malamuth and Donnerstein, eds., *Pornography and Sexual Aggression.*

21. Abbey, "Sex Differences in Attributions for Friendly Behavior: Do Males Misperceive Females' Friendliness?": 830; D. N. Lipton, E. C. McDonnel, and R. M. McFall, "Heterosexual Perception in Rapists," *Journal of Consulting and Clinical Psychology* 55, no. 1 (1987): 17.

22. Michael S. Kimmel, "Clarence, William, Iron Mike, Tailhook, Senator Pack-

wood, Spur Posse, Magic . . . and Us," in Buchwald, Fletcher, and Roth, eds., *Transforming a Rape Culture*, 124.

23. N. M. Malamuth, "Rape Proclivity Among Males," *Journal of Social Issues* 37 (1981): 138.

24. Virginia Greendlinger and Donn Byrne, "Coerceive Sexual Fantasies of College Men and Predictors of Self-reported Likelihood to Rape and Overt Sexual Aggression," *Journal of Sex Research* 23 (1987): 1.

25. Warshaw, *I Never Called It Rape.*

26. Susan Forward and Joan Torres, *Men Who Hate Women and the Women Who Love Them,* (New York: Bantam Books, 1986).

27. Elizabeth Powell, "I Thought You Didn't Mind," in Buchwald, Fletcher, and Roth, eds., *Transforming a Rape Culture*, 116.

28. E. Sandra Byers, Barbara L. Giles, and Dorothy L. Price, "Definiteness and Effectiveness of Women's Responses to Unwanted Sexual Advances," *Basic and Applied Social Psychology* 8, no. 4 (1987): 321.

29. "Rape: The Macho View," quoting the research of D. L. Mosher and R. D. Anderson, *Psychology Today* 21 (April 1987), 12.

30. As described by Charlene L. Muehlenhard and Jennifer L. Schrag, "Nonviolent Sexual Coercion," in Andrea Parrot and Laurie Gechhofer, eds., *Acquaintance Rape: The Hidden Crime* (New York: John Wiley and Sons, 1991), 120.

31. Judith M. Siegel et al., "Resistance to Sexual Assault: Who Resists and What Happens?" *American Journal of Public Health* 79, no. 1 (January 1989): 27.

32. Joyce Levine-McCombie and Mary P. Koss, "Acquaintance Rape: Effective Avoidance Strategies," *Psychology of Women Quarterly* 10 (1986): 311.

33. Siegel et al. "Resistance to Sexual Assault."

34. Pauline B. Bart and Patricia H. O'Brien, *Stopping Rape* (New York: Pergamon Press, 1985).

35. Charlene L. Muehlenhard, Debra E. Friedman, and Celeste M. Thomas, "Is Date Rape Justifiable?" *Psychology of Woman Quarterly* 9, no. 3 (1985): 297.

36. Madhubuti, "On Becoming Anti-Rapist," in Buchwald, Fletcher, and Roth, eds., *Transforming a Rape Culture*, 174–5.

37. Siegel et al., "Resistance to Sexual Assault."

38. Linda Braswell, *Quest for Respect* (Ventura, Calif.: Pathfinder Publishing of California, 1990), 25.

39. Braswell, *Quest for Respect,* 12.

8

Responding to Other Intrusions

For of course, when someone new approaches us, we are all caution; we take that person's measure.[1]
— *DORIS LESSING*

The phone rings. Susan answers it.

"Hello."

"Hello, there. This is a friend of yours."

Her heart pounds. Tentatively, she says, "Who is speaking?"

"It's Gary."

She realizes she's been holding her breath.

"Oh, Gary! You scared me."

You scared me. In our sexual jungle, the least uncertainty can become a threat. Hearing the unidentified voice of a man—*of half the human race*—can represent terrifying possibilities to an American woman answering her telephone.

Persuading, Intruding, and Coercing

A person can try to get sexual pleasure from another person in a variety of ways—with or without consent, directly, or indirectly, by force or peacefully. When John wants to be more sexual and Mary refuses, John has a number of choices. He can try to *persuade* Mary with words or nonforceful actions, such as touching her in an arousing way. If she isn't willing to go further, he can stop trying and use some indirect and harmless way to get sexual satisfaction, such as fantasy or masturbation. John could attempt to coerce Mary by threats or by force. Or he could find another partner.

There is a great difference between persuasion and coercion. "Please," "C'mon," "Why not?" fall in the realm of persuasion, while "Put out or get out of the car!" falls in the area of coercion. But some people never even try to obtain direct sexual contact, by persuasion or any other means. Rather than asking for a date or approaching a sex partner directly, they seek unusual and indirect sexual outlets for gratification. Many sex offenders intrude upon your space without attempting to persuade or to coerce you. Obscene phone callers break into your auditory space. An exhibitionist trespasses on your visual space. A voyeur or Peeping Tom invades your personal privacy.

You have a right to be free from sexual intrusion. Noncoercive intrusion is invasion of your physical surroundings or your psychological space without your consent. Coercion occurs when someone compels you to do something through strong force, such as threat of physical harm or physical power. "I'll slit your throat if you move" is such a threat; holding someone down so that she can't move is using physical power.

Sometimes people intrude unintentionally, as Rachel did one night last year when she entered the rest room at the movies. For about two seconds, she wondered about the strange little sinks that sat so low to the floor. When she realized she was in the men's room, she bolted out. Had anyone been there, Rachel would have accidentally intruded upon his physical and psychological space, but there was no coercion involved. (Indeed, she was eager to leave the situation.) It is possible to intrude without coercing someone, but it is not possible to coerce someone sexually without intrusion.

How can we decide which kind of intrusion is more serious than another? One way might be to consider how physically close the intruder gets to the other person, setting the degrees of physical intrusion on a continuum.

Degrees of Sexual Intrusion and Coercion

The following list ranks sexual acts according to their physical intrusiveness:

0. There is no intrusion or coercion: partners consent to all sexual activities.

1. Intrusion is beginning, but the intruder's intentions are uncertain and he is physically distant: leering or ogling.

2. The intruder's actions are clearly sexual, and he enters the auditory or visual space of another: sexual gestures or sexual remarks without consent.

3. An anonymous intruder invades the other's auditory space: obscene phone calling.

4. The intruder further invades the other's physical or visual space with clear sexual intent: exhibitionism (exhibiting one's genitals without the other's consent) or voyeurism (watching another's private sexual experiences from a hidden vantage point.)

5. The intruder physically coerces another person into contact with *nonsexual* body areas (such as a hand on the arm, an arm around the waist.)

6. The intruder physically coerces another person into contact with *sexual* areas of that person's body but does not rape: touching of buttocks, breasts, or genitals without consent.

7. The intruder coerces another person into sexual penetration without using physical force: misuse of authority over the victim, strong verbal threats or pressures, or administering a substance to the other for the purpose of preventing resistance. (In some states any or all of these acts constitute rape.)

8. The intruder physically coerces the other into oral, anal, or vaginal penetration, through sexual intercourse or by insertion of objects.

The legal definition of rape differs from state to state. Although the list classifies sexual acts in order of their *physical* intrusiveness, the level of seriousness to the victim also varies because of other factors. Most people would rather have somebody put an arm around the waist (5) than be subjected to the sight of a stranger's genitalia (4). The person committing the offense is also important. A woman may feel that a fourteen-year-old neighbor standing in her yard at night is less threatening than the stranger who cruises the alleys, looking for a lighted window.

All of the acts in 1–8 above are uninvited. They involve sex without consent. They do not involve verbal *persuasion*; they violate another person's sexual privacy. Although the experts do not agree totally on what constitutes healthy, normal sex, all agree that it occurs only between consenting adults. It involves no coercion.

Coercion of Men

It may seem at first glance that men are not victimized by any of the coercive acts in the above list. But nearly one in seven little boys suffers sexual abuse, sometimes from women perpetrators. Exploitation of boys is a serious national concern. Males victimized in childhood can become sex offenders in adulthood. Mary Calderone, M.D., former executive director of the Sex Information and Education Council of the United States, says we must educate now for sexual health if we are to stop the chain of sexual abuse. "Time is of the essence," she warns, "for the next generation of sexually violent criminals is already in the ranks."[2]

Men can also suffer from sexual harassment. As we saw in the last chapter, as many as one in ten rapes are rapes of men. Those who are never personally victimized may suffer, even so, from the exploitation of others. Intrusion and coercion of a woman involves every man in our society. If a man accidentally entered a *women's* rest room, a woman who misinterpreted his presence could create an unpleasant episode with the police. Because of the terrifying sexual climate in this country, innocent men are vulnerable to accusations, and they should be as eager as women to correct this situation.

Would Assertiveness Help?

Because some intrusive and coercive acts are quite serious and harmful—either physically or to one's job or school success—no one can give you simple advice about precisely how to handle every case. You might have to respond with silence, running away, or even violence in dealing with a particular sexual intruder. You should be aware, however, that people who exploit others often count on their victims' compliance. They frequently fantasize about being turned on by a passive victim. Their power needs have been formed in a culture that links sexual conquest to domination. There will be times when you could speak assertively to a potential exploiter who is counting on your passivity, and you might reverse the script in the perpetrator's mind.

Just as bacteria cannot multiply without nourishment, sexual victimization can happen only where the climate is right. When a society subtly suggests that an attractive woman should be passive and an attractive man should be pushy and aggressive, this attitude reinforces the climate of sexual violence. If you don't think violence against women is a part of our everyday life, consider the fact that every fifteen seconds another American woman is beaten up by a man.

The Importance of Using Your Own Judgment

You can learn effective responses to some forms of sexual intrusion, which increase your repertoire in situations where you are able to react. This does not mean there's a solution to every problem, or that you should check with a book before using your instincts. You should never apply advice automatically. You may need alternatives to consider, perhaps ideas for responding that never occurred to you, but nothing can replace your own evaluation of the circumstances. Do not ignore your judgment, even if you're scared. If someone says or does something sexually pressuring or seeks to intrude upon you, listen to your inner voice, your vibes and intuitive feelings. They are important. Then, if assertion seems appropriate, be prepared to say something.

Uninvited Sexual Staring

I read a newspaper article that described a male police decoy arresting another man in a public rest room. One of the charges was "making significant eye contact" with the policeman. And in the early eighties, in the college where I was teaching, the new harassment policy mentioned ogling as a form of harassment.

It's risky to accuse another person of just looking at someone the wrong way. Few things are as open to misinterpretation. It's hard to define a facial expression. People who feel scared, wronged, and defensive may read all kinds of unintended motives into a look. Still, a look can be both frightening and intimidating. At a milder level, it can be annoying and distracting. If you think women are overly sensitive about how men look at them, at least try to be open to the possibility that looks can scare someone. Although you might absolutely love it if someone stared at you with sexual interest, somebody else might find it ominous. There is so much confusion about sexual intentions that we need to consider where looking leaves off and ogling or leering begins.

It's impossible to make an absolute rule about what constitutes inappropriate looking; the boundaries keep shifting. Even in our country, staring is more accepted in some groups than in others. What's all right in downtown Manhattan may not be acceptable in Salt Lake City. All of us need to learn early in life what is sexually proper so that we don't have to stop and think about what to do in every situation. In the absence of this early learning, I am going to try to offer some guidelines about what sexual staring, ogling, or leering comprises.

Appreciative and Admiring Glances

If someone looks at you in a sexual manner, he may intend no offense. If you happen to have a gorgeous figure or build, even in your smart business suit you may receive occasional admiring or sexually interested glances. How long can a legitimate look last? In my opinion, if a person is looking at someone and the other person knows it, a look that lasts two or three seconds is probably not a leer or ogling. Looking at someone for a longer time—if the person is aware of it—is called *staring*, and if it is sexual, *leering* or *ogling*. All three can be intimidating if unwelcome. People should be able to expect restraint and good manners, and when a person catches himself staring for more than a few seconds, he's supposed to gain control quickly and look elsewhere. It's also inappropriate to gawk at another person's body; in our culture, you're expected to look at the face of the person to whom you're speaking.

You could be looking at someone who has no idea you're looking. That is usually not considered an offense in a public place. If you have a terrific crush on someone and you're sitting behind her in a meeting, it's fun to feast your eyes. But if you were sitting directly facing her, it would become an affront.

What You Are Wearing

Clothes never cause anyone to use sexual force on another person. You have a right to wear anything you want. Are clothes meaningless, then? They may contribute to others' inclination to stare at you if they deliberately emphasize your sexual characteristics—for example, wearing a blouse that reveals much of your breasts, or a very short skirt. Men who wear very tight pants may also attract attention. Most people associate women with seductive clothes.

This comment from a woman could create an outrage in some camps. Am I blaming women for other people's behavior? No, I am saying that clothing can draw attention. Whatever the female intends, there is research to show that men—even men who would never coerce a woman—may think the woman is somehow advertising her interest in having sex. Most women find this puzzling.

I especially worry about young teenagers who dress in ways that are perceived by males as seductive. They may think that the latest sexy fashion is great. But does everyone who notices them understand that although they're making a fashion statement, they're not necessarily issuing a sexual invitation? Those who wear seductive clothes may attract attention, but they still have the same sexual rights as those who do not. *Clothes do not give sexual consent; only words and clear actions can tell someone you're sexually available.* In practical terms, however, when you're surrounded by people who are confused about your rights, and you don't want them to leer at you, you'd be smart to keep that in mind when you choose your clothes. They may leer anyway, but you are acting with greater awareness.

Aside from unintentional intrusion, some people stare at the breasts, buttocks, or genital area of another person inappropriately long or give the "bouncing eyebrow" kind of sexual leer. They seem to know what they are doing. This kind of staring from a stranger is usually more threatening, particularly to a woman in a rape-prone culture like ours. Men, not fearing sexual harm, may find a woman's leering complimentary or exciting. Or, if the man thinks the leering woman is bizarre, he may pass her off as a kook, but he is usually not afraid. Being the object of leering can also be threatening if it's from a person who has power over you at work or school or from an acquaintance whom you do not trust.

Brain Wiring

It has escaped the notice of very few people that men seem to respond sexually to what they see. This applies both to heterosexual and to gay men. Looking at women's bodies, heterosexual men often show more interest than the average woman does when looking at men. Gay men also respond with excitement to the sight of other men's bodies. This tendency to be visually stimulated could be cultural, because of our teaching girls and women that looking isn't nice or discreet. The difference could be exaggerated by the porn industry. Men often report sexual fantasies that include visual images of women's bodies; women more often fantasize about sexual feelings.

Research in the last few years reveals clear differences between male and female brains. Some evidence suggests that male brains may be "wired" to become more aroused by sights.[3] Our culture, no doubt, encourages males to look, but it may also have been an evolutionary advantage for men to be turned on by looking.

Voyeurs (Peeping Toms) are usually men. Very few women's magazines capitalize on nudity. Women can undeniably enjoy and become aroused by looking, but the tendency is ordinarily stronger in men. Many men say that they find it very difficult not to look at a sexually exciting woman. I mention this tendency because we need to differentiate between sexual interest in what we see and staring to the point of intrusion. I'm acquainted with some very respectful heterosexual men, not one of whom ignores an attractive woman without some effort. Leering goes beyond this point. If you want to attract someone across a room, and you stare at that person, you wouldn't call it leering; you might even call it flirting. Leering is unwelcome.

Should You Speak Up to Someone Who Is Leering at You?

If you are the object of leering, should you say anything? Most people would advise you to leave well enough alone and ignore it, especially if the intruder is a stranger. Your remarks might be taken as a come-on or make you more conspicuous to him. He might give up leering at you if you refuse to respond.

But maybe someone you know stares at your buttocks, breasts, or pelvic area in such a way that you feel you must say something and you believe you would be safe to do so. A colleague may gape and ogle at you even at meetings, where you become embarrassed and uncomfortable. No one can keep his professional dignity when someone distracts him in this way. You could make an I-statement to the person in private: "I don't know if you realize it, but you're staring at me. It's really distracting." Or: "I feel very uncomfortable when you keep staring at me. I want you to stop."

At that point, a considerate person stops looking. But there is no guarantee that a hard-core ogler will do so. He may not admit that it's happening, or he might even accuse you of oversensitivity. Again and again we see that people who are sexually intrusive hold distorted ideas about what they're doing and whether the victim likes it. Very rarely, an ogler may be so hostile that he *enjoys* making you uncomfortable.

If this leering happens at work or at school, it could be illegal sexual harassment. What to do about that is addressed in Chapter 6.

Uninvited Sexual Comments

What kinds of sexual comments are intrusive and which are complimentary? Many people are frustrated by having to squelch sincere compliments and affectionate remarks because someone might mistake them as inappropriate or sexist.

How a person interprets a compliment depends on the context. "My, don't you look lovely!" is not a sexual comment in itself, unless the nonverbal message from the person is sexual. If a person stares at your pelvic area while telling you look lovely, for example, that is sexual. It is also improper to compliment a person's looks when she's engaged in some professional task. This happened to Brenda, a single mother who has worked hard to attain an executive position in her company. Brenda's a bit nervous because today is her first presentation before the entire executive group. She is an attractive woman who has struggled to overcome sexist attitudes and feel like a competent professional. She prepared carefully for today's meeting. As she organizes her papers, just before she gets up to speak, Gene leans over with a wink and says, "Baby, you look fantastic!" Her heart sinks, and some of her old doubts about herself come back. She tries to shut out his leering grin while he looks up and down her body as she rises to present herself at her professional best.

Such an uninvited sexual comment can be a jolt to a person who doesn't expect it. Yelling, "Look at the jugs on that broad!" is a sexual comment, an unwelcome joke about a woman's body. Experts note that intrusions such as sexual yelling happen more often in violent societies. Though a few women still encourage such remarks, people have begun to express anger about them. Uninvited remarks about someone's sexual qualities are a form of sexual intrusion; everyone should have a right not to have his body commented upon without his consent.

A related indignity occurs with surprising frequency on college campuses. Pam describes the typical situation:

I was walking across the triangle to my math class. As I approached one of the dormitories, I heard these voices yelling. "She's a five!" one of them said. "Hell, no! She's a two!" another guy hollered. I realized—they are rating my appearance! Some of the others were yelling too. I felt so humiliated that I stumbled and almost fell. Now I walk ten minutes out of my way to avoid that house.

Few people like being talked about as if they were mere objects, even when the remarks seem complimentary. You can yell about your admiration for a car, but a human being has feelings. Fortunately, a number of colleges and universities are attempting to educate students about these actions. Comments about their bodies may also offend men. A very handsome man may tire of hearing what he views as irrelevant remarks. He is probably not frightened by them, but when someone ignores what he is saying or doing and just looks at his body it can frustrate or embarrass him.

Once in a while a certain female entertainer responds with a smile to jokes about her enormous breasts. You might also find yourself flattered when someone—even a stranger—whistles at you from a construction site or a dormitory, or otherwise comments about your looks. Unfortunately, however, your smiling acceptance of these actions may be misinterpreted. You're living in a rape culture. It's risky to imply that it's tolerable or even flattering for a stranger to remark about the sexual aspects of your body.

This mixed message about intrusion's being complimentary even extends to violent actions. In St. Louis, a recent trial involved two law students. In the bar where they met, the man had bitten the woman, a stranger, on the buttocks. She took him to court. His comment was, "What's wrong with her? She doesn't know how to take a compliment!" If he'd bitten her on the nose, his act would have been perceived accurately as assault. Because it was her buttock, in our society there may be just the slightest doubt—was it complimentary? Won't boys be boys? Fortunately, the judge did not think so.

What to Say to Uninvited Sexual Comments

There is obviously no hard-and-fast rule about when to respond to sexual remarks. The old wisdom of not speaking to intrusive strangers is still valid. If a stranger is inappropriate enough to comment on your body without your consent, this intruder might be more likely to intrude in other ways. If you need a way to respond to someone you know, though, and you think he might respond, you could make an I-statement:

"Maybe you meant it as a compliment, but to me it is very intrusive when you comment about my body." (If this approach does not work, the offender may be so domineering and aggressive that he enjoys your discomfort.)

"I'm hurt and embarrassed when you yell out numbers to rate the way I look."

"I am getting really irritated with these remarks about my appearance."

You could escalate your assertion:

"I'm fed up with having to listen to what *you think* about *my body.*"

Or you may decide that sounds too textbook and just say, "Knock it off!" Such a sharp retort may work; some people won't respond to a civilized request and have to be treated with anger. But "Knock it off!" is not specific, and *if* your goal is to teach the offender about the effect of the remark on you, you would not want to respond that way. Don't underestimate the power of revealing your emotional reaction to someone who is capable of change. Letting others know that they are really causing you pain can be educational to some violators. Hard-core offenders may not care, but borderline offenders may learn from your reactions. Your negative experience contradicts what the boys are telling each other: that sex and scoring are all in good fun.

You could yell and holler and cuss at the people who make the remarks, too, but that kind of aggression might even encourage them. But don't squelch all of your aggressive retorts—just try to be aware of your options. Some people would like it if they got a rise out of you. So you're already in a difficult situation. You have to try to figure out what would be most discouraging to this particular person.

But remember, it is not your fault if you cannot solve this problem. It's the other person who is intruding upon your rights.

Harassing comments at school or work are often illegal, depending upon the circumstances. Check Chapter 6 and the Appendix for information.

Obscene Phone Calls

Scaring people through obscene telephone messages is against the law, but it is disturbingly common. For the last ten years I have informally polled my students to see who has received obscene calls. Through 1985, 95 percent of the women and 2 percent of the men in my classes had received at least one call. In the years since then the numbers have risen to 99.8 percent of the women and approximately 5 percent of the men.

Unfortunately, there is very little research about obscene phone callers, whose intrusions have been regarded as rather trivial compared to other sex offenses. In a context that includes something extremely serious like rape, people tend to view other sex offenses as less important. But we need to respect the terror of a person who, in a society filled with sex crimes, is subjected to threatening voices in her own living or working space.

We pay little attention to *men* who receive obscene calls. When I ask how many men students have felt afraid or been intimidated by receiving obscene calls, very few raise their hands. There is a snickering, comical attitude in the classroom about these calls, which sometimes come from men and sometimes from women. Almost never does a man say the call scared him, although it may have and he felt it was unmanly to admit it in class. When I ask the women how many were scared by the calls they received, almost every one raises her hand.

Who is making these calls? Some offenders are young teenage pranksters. Others are adults with a compulsive need to make calls, usually while masturbating. A common kind of obscene phone call is made by an ex-boyfriend in retaliation for being rejected. Women in such a case should be extra cautious; ex-boyfriends also commit a high number of acquaintance rapes and can become dangerous stalkers. (See Chapter 7.)

Responding to the Obscene Phone Caller

Should you assert yourself with the obscene caller? Here are some suggestions:

1. Strongly consider not responding at all to an obscene caller. By talking, you could legitimize the call and encourage it. This person does not deserve the courtesy of a conversation. He is an abuser who is violating you. Hang up.

2. Consider carefully whether you want to say or do something punitive or painful, such as insulting the caller. Police often advise victims to blow a whistle in the caller's ear or to hang up. There are no surveys of obscene callers to find out what they find discouraging. I have some reservations about doing anything that might anger an unknown person who may have your name and address. If you plan to take a more assertive stand than hanging up, you may be reassured to know that retaliation by an obscene caller is rare. But it has happened.

3. If you have a problem with a caller who keeps dialing you again within a few minutes, you can take the phone off the hook. There's no reward in that beeping busy signal for the caller. You can also screen your calls with an answering device before picking up the phone. An occasional intruder just fills up the recording with obscene messages.

4. Be aware of the common ploys used by callers. One is to impersonate someone taking a survey. This person gradually asks more and more personal questions. Another ploy is to make a preliminary call impersonating a policeman who is tracking an obscene caller. Police do not do this kind of work by phone. If you get one of these calls you should hang up.

5. Some women have used another technique with obscene callers: tell them they need help and give them the name of Sex Addicts Anonymous or another counseling group. It's tempting—just think, all over America millions of obscene callers would get a referral for help instead of an opportunity to scare someone! But as our society is becoming more violent, I would be concerned that your referral might possibly hook the caller into having an even greater interest, or greater anger, toward you, rather than just going on with another call. Again, only you can be responsible for evaluating whether to say anything to an obscene phone caller.

Although most callers are not likely to become violent, I have known an obscene phone caller to commit acquaintance rape. The obscene caller is already moving down the scale of intrusion and coercion that we saw at the beginning of this chapter. A repeated obscene phone caller is willing to get sexual gratification out of frightening another person anonymously, rather than from a real sexual partner. Such a person is confused and—while he may be too passive to take physical action—should be viewed seriously as a sexual intruder.

6. New telephone options promise to decrease if not prevent obscene phone calls. You can ask the phone company to give you the services that block calls, identify callers, and other protective alternatives. If you cannot afford these methods and have been receiving obscene or threatening calls, the telephone company will usually put a trap on your line which will keep a log for them of who is calling you. You can then file a complaint with the police and the phone company will turn over its records. New possibilities are arising every year. Call and find out what your options are.

7. Many women list their phone numbers under their last names and first initials to avoid identifying themselves as females. Some callers have caught on to this trick. In addition, of course, a temporary or permanent unlisted number is an option.

Exhibitionists and Voyeurs

Flashers

Every city and college campus has its exhibitionists. Exhibitionists expose their genitals to strangers without consent. "Flashing" is the most common cause of arrest of any sexual offense in the United States. In fact, exhibitionists seem to have a need to get caught and often expose themselves in situations that involve the most risk of being apprehended.

We make a lot of jokes about male flashers. In one restaurant, I've seen a picture viewed from the back of a teddy bear in a raincoat, holding the coat open and flashing. It's obviously intended to be cute and funny. The other art on the wall is pleasant and suitable. We laugh at flasher cartoons, because the humor catches us before we realize what we're doing. But victims of exhibitionists do not laugh.

In a country like ours where violent sex crimes happen often, women are frightened by seeing an exhibitionist. Victims of flashers report a variety of emotions afterwards, but some are so afraid that they even stop going out to their regular activities. Up to half of those who have seen an exhibitionist later report fears of going out alone.

There are females with a tendency to exhibitionism. But unless they are psychotic and do something like running nude and screaming through the streets, such women usually are not taken seriously. Our society encourages females to expose as much of their bodies as legally possible; and it encourages males to believe that seeing more of a woman is something to be desired—to be pushed for, in fact. These opposing messages cause many men to discount the seriousness of this crime to women.

Exhibitionists always try to surprise you, so it's difficult to be prepared to respond. Should you comment? One woman of my acquaintance suggests greeting the exhibitionist with the sardonic reply "I've seen better at Woolworth's." However, remember you are dealing with a sexual intruder. He is invading your sexual privacy, thereby demonstrating that he has some sexual confusion. Although exhibitionism usually develops in a passive man, occasionally a dangerous flasher emerges. It is probably best to make no comment to an exhibitionist until research tells us what such men perceive as a turnoff.

Your nonverbal behavior toward an exhibitionist may count, too. To the extent that you can disregard the behavior and leave the situation, you would seem to remove the reward. It may not matter if you show shock, however; Masters, Johnson, and Kolodny list only two cases where an exhibitionist hurt someone, and in each case he claimed it made him angry when the victim did not react sufficiently.[4]

Voyeurs

A voyeur is a person who gets sexual gratification from spying on people who are undressing, nude, or engaging in sexual activity. He may do this by looking through windows, heat vents, intricate mirror arrangements, or even cameras. Voyeurs have trouble relating to women and they sometimes commit more serious crimes. Rather than committing the offense in a public place like the exhibitionist, the voyeur enters your private physical *and* psychological space. He is a serious sexual intruder.

I've occasionally heard of women who attempted the "paradoxical intervention" technique when discovering a voyeur. One woman opened the door and loudly invited him in. I would not advise attempting to interact with a voyeur. If you discover a voyeur, your first job is to ensure your safety. Lock your doors and windows; close your drapes. Call the police. Then call a neighbor if possible. The odds are that you will be safe; *most* voyeurs do no physical harm.

Protecting Yourself from Stalkers

A young friend confided to me that someone had stolen her driver's license and was calling her apartment frequently. She even had considerable evidence that someone had been *in* her apartment, although she could not figure out how he did it. She received phone calls from this person in which he told her how much he cared for her. She called me for advice. I told her to call the police first, but she also told me something that alerted me to a change that she needed to make in herself. She naturally wanted to try old responses for this new situation. She said, "When he calls, should I try again to explain how much this bothers me, and how I'd really like him to quit?" I said, "No, absolutely not. He is already distorting your interest in him. A conversation might give him food for fantasy." However, when he called she wasn't able to resist pleading with him to stop. He increased his contacts with her until she had to move. He might have continued anyway. She still is not sure that she's safe from him.

I'm hearing about more and more people being stalked by some angry or romantically obsessed person. Stalking is not necessarily a sexual crime, but it can be the precursor of rape, assault, or murder. It appears to be on the increase. Most states either have laws against stalking, or are in the process of enacting them. To be clear, the laws must add several definitions. Missouri Law, for example, breaks down the offense into Aggravated Stalking and Stalking:[5]

> *Aggravated Stalking is purposefully and repeatedly harassing or following, with the intent of harassing or actually harassing another person and the making of a credible threat that has or intends to place the individual being stalked in reasonable fear of death or serious injury. Stalking is the crime of purposefully and repeatedly harassing or following with the intent of harassing another person. A credible threat is one that has the intent of causing the person who is the target to reasonably fear for his or her safety and must be against the life or be a threat to cause physical injury to a person. Harassing is the engaging in of conduct that is*

directed at a specific individual that has or serves no legitimate purpose but causes a reasonable individual to suffer emotional distress and actually does cause substantial emotional damage to the individual. For either of the crimes, a Court Order of Protection can be obtained.

The stalker who has focused on you romantically presents a scary dilemma. A normal person can take no for an answer. If someone you liked were clearly disinterested, you might call or write once or twice to make your case, but unless you were obsessed, you would not follow this person around. Some stalkers know that you do not like being stalked, but the romantic preoccupations of others cloud their perceptions of your feelings. They are distorting reality; they often feel they have a right to you as a partner. They are obsessed. Like rapists, they have a sense of entitlement. They are powerfully distorting their rights to your psychological and physical space, despite clear messages that they are unwelcome. Remember, some imprisoned rapists even think their black-and-blue victims loved it. We are living in a society in which individuals make extremely confused judgments about others' intentions. Stalking is a hostile and disturbed act, and you are correct to be very concerned.

As with all the advice in this book, you must use your own judgment. But be aware of your rights. Call the police; check your state's laws on stalking. You do not have to make an official police report unless you want to, but it is something you should strongly consider. Weigh carefully how you should proceed, get advice from more than one trusted person as well as from the police. In some cases you may want to consider living elsewhere for a while, changing locks, changing your itinerary and habits, buying mace or pepper spray, and other safety measures. In Colorado, a pilot project requires stalkers to wear electronic ankle bracelets that trigger an alarm if the stalker goes near his victim. If you have a women's self-help center of any kind in your community, you may want to call it and ask for further advice.

Remember, just because a restraining order is in effect does not mean you are safe. Continue to take precautions. Some stalkers just give up after a while.

Treatment for the Sexual Intruder

Voyeurism, compulsive obscene phone calling, and exhibitionism can be viewed as sexual addictions—compulsive sexual behaviors. But they result in a vicious cycle of embarrassment, fear, and self-hatred in the offender. There is treatment for these addictions. See the Appendix for places to find therapists or groups that help with sexual addiction.

Reporting the Sexual Intruder

These offenses are against the law. You should report them immediately to your local police. The police generally treat victims with respect, but sometimes may not take these crimes as seriously as the victim deserves. Do not let that deter you. There is clear experimental evidence that, after encountering an event that is *very* serious, individuals tend to react less to *moderately* serious occurrences. ("With all these rapes, lady, how bad can a little old flasher be?" "A phone call? Aw, those guys never hurt you. Go on and go to sleep.") Don't go along with that attitude. If you feel that a police officer's treatment of your complaint is demeaning or condescending, you can always make a complaint to that person's superior. If someone intrudes upon your sexual privacy, expect the police to take your report seriously. You are less a victim; you become a survivor when you take action to help yourself cope. Get emotional support from others who agree with your perception.

You cannot absolutely prevent sexual intruders from attempting to get their sexual gratification from you. But you can be alert, aware, and courageous enough to speak out against them when this is safe for you.

Which Intrusions Have You Experienced?

Check below which of these sexually intrusive experiences have ever been directed at you. Stay in the column for your gender, Male or Female. Then rate the amount of fear you felt at the time, with 0 being no fear and 10 being panic:

TABLE 8-1

0   1   2   3   4   5   6   7   8   9   10

	Male	Female	Fear Level
Heard sexual remark from stranger (could be comments on your body) # of times you recall:			
Received obscene phone call # of times you recall:			
Observed an exhibitionist # of times you recall: Where were you?			
Discovered a voyeur, or anyone trying to observe you in any private situation:			

Notes

1. Doris Lessing, *The Memoirs of a Survivor* (New York: Bantam Books, 1976), 31.

2. Carol Cassell and Pamela Wilson, *Sexuality Education: A Resource Book* (New York: Garland, 1989), 7.

3. J. J. Furedy et. al., "Sex Differences in Small-Magnitude Heart-Rate Responses to Sexual and Infant-related Stimuli: A Psychophysiological Approach," *Physiology and Behavior* 46 (1989): 903–905, reported in Katharine Blick Hoyenga and Kermit T. Hoyenga, *Gender-Related Differences: Origins and Outcomes* (Boston: Allyn and Bacon, 1993), 383.

4. Masters, Johnson, and Kolodny, *Human Sexuality*, 423.

5. Interpretation of Missouri Statute 455.0101–455.085, by *Meramec College Police Campuswatch,* Spring–Summer 1994.

Part IV

How to Speak Up for Your Society

9

Searching for
the Causes

> . . . it is the basic taboos . . .
> against "unthinkable" behavior
> that keep the social system in balance.[1]
> —MARGARET MEAD

So far this book has shown you the necessity to talk back in the face of sexual pressure and become sexually assertive for your personal safety. Now we will consider what you can say to protect your society. But why should you have to bother? What has happened that we find ourselves living with such sexual fears? What are the major causes, and can we control any of them?

There is no question that our sexual problems have complex origins. Many of the causes can be traced to family dysfunction, exploitative influences in the media, drugs, and shifting values. Most of these issues are beyond the scope of this book. However, there are some reasons for our sexual problems that we have largely ignored and over which we could have some influence.

Whatever Happened to Moral Outrage?

Moral outrage has the ring of an old-fashioned, rigid idea. When millions of people watch vicious acts committed against their own kind, day after day, their senses become dulled. Americans have lost sight of what is out-of-bounds. And we calmly accept things now that once caused offense, including not only extreme violence, but also very subtle forms of sexual exploitation.

Millions of viewers sit enthralled watching perpetrators and their victims on television. Such shows explore topics like "Child molesters and the women who love them." Encouraged by a seemingly sincere host or hostess, the abuser and abused discuss their traumatic experience with all the emotion of a couple of friends getting over a little tiff. This courteous treatment gives the impression that sexual exploitation is not really serious; after all, aren't perpetrators and victims sitting there discussing their ordeal as total equals, as if all were forgiven? A simple confession seems to make everything okay.

Why are we not outraged that incest survivors are encouraged to sit and chat in public with the fathers who took their innocence? One rationale is that offenders deserve sympathy. They have often been victimized themselves, and they certainly deserve treatment. But some things, as Margaret Mead says in the quotation that heads this chapter, must be *unthinkable*. Otherwise people believe that they can act on even their most forbidden impulses.

Our culture has even brainwashed its own lawmakers. "But if you can't rape your wife, who can you rape?" This comment was made by a male California state senator to a group lobbying for a bill that would make it illegal for a man to force his wife to have sexual intercourse. Raping one's wife was legal in all states until one woman in California began the lobbying effort. And it is not only male legislators who encourage rape. A female state representative in Missouri, defending her statement that some women ask to be raped, replied, "Gosh, you can't blame a guy—that's their chemical makeup."

Do the media—films, television, printed matter—contribute to these distorted views on rape? The way our society represents sex in the media is often harmful. We have documented evidence of this fact. Because of the current depths to which our standards have sunk, the pressure for government censorship is increasing. Just censoring the media for explicit sex, however, does not get at the real problems.

Can the Media Cause Sexual Violence?

A 12-year-old boy in Rhode Island had seen a television program about a gang rape on a pool table. He forced a 10-year-old girl onto his pool table and sexually assaulted her while other children watched. A few viewers, like that boy, actually copy some of the horrid acts that we use to entertain ourselves. But our greatest worry is not whether viewers will directly *imitate* what they see. Only a few people who watch violence actually imitate it. Even more alarming are the powerful *attitude* changes documented repeatedly by research. In slasher films seen by thousands of American males, men stab, rape, beat, torture, decapitate, scalp, cut with saws, burn, shoot with nail guns, or drill women with an electric drill. Does watching these films change something mentally in the viewers? The answer is yes.

Before looking at the research on how the media influence sex in our society, let's take a moment to address the major accusation leveled at anyone who wants to improve the media.

Censorship and the Rape Culture

Censorship is official suppression before a work is published or put on public display. Pickets, boycotts, and other forms of protest are not violations of the First Amendment; they are legal. Citizen pressure is not censorship. Without organized efforts to push for their civil rights, African Americans and women might still be unable to vote in parts of the United States.

The First Amendment of our Bill of Rights says, in part, "Congress shall make no law . . . abridging the freedom of speech, or of the press . . . " A few exceptions have been made to this principle, such as saying something that causes a clear and present danger (like yelling "fire" in a crowded theater), or saying something that incites people to engage in other lawless actions. Saying something libelous is also illegal, as is obscenity—which no one so far has been able to define.

Our freedom of expression allows the media to show things that can hurt people. Making another exception to the First Amendment is very serious matter, but we must face the threats in today's media in order to find other solutions that might work. It is not just zealots who want to improve TV and movies. Even certain professionals have become so unnerved over the incriminating research that they have been tempted to advocate some kind of regulations. Some feminists consider violent and degrading pornography to be a way of teaching rape—a violation of women's civil rights—and have pressed for legislation to ban it. Sandra Campbell, a consultant on children and violence, writes that " . . . there must be a balance between individuals' rights to freely express their sadistic fantasies and the right of women, for example, to live without threat of violence."[2]

However, censorship brings with it some problems. For one thing, it would not guarantee that people will form healthy attitudes toward sex. It brings the risk of extreme government suppression, such as banning all books that even mention sex. Furthermore, if we censor, where do we draw the line in what is legal? Will some people want to outlaw pictures that help women find lumps in their breasts? Or discussions of condoms as a disease-preventive measure? If we did regulate the harmful material in the media we would have to have some method of deciding what to include. Some of the most damaging material is not rated X. Our society is more worried that its children will see someone making love on TV than killing someone. Censorship is a very complicated issue.

We need to raise the consciousness of our entire society toward the kinds of media that can cause sexual harm. Even if authorities did not censor entertainment that had been proved harmful, outraged citizens could bring about change. Our pressure on the media could change their definition of appropriate sexual relationships. There is such a thing as good taste and good judgment. Insulting Blacks, Jews, or Hispanics is legal but no longer acceptable in the media. Public disapproval is much more effective when people voluntarily decide to take action rather than invite heavy-handed government intervention.

The Findings of Government Commissions

There is not space here to document all the research showing harm from violence on TV. Among these data is the surgeon general's "Report on Television Violence," which at long last concluded that people could actually learn to be violent from the mass media.

Sex in the media takes a variety of forms, not all of which do demonstrable harm. The impact of sex in the media is not a simple topic. Not everything has a single cause, and that's why we need an educated population. Single-cause thinking ("What's wrong with this country is that other people don't go to my church") misses the complexity of the issue and divides people. Another elementary viewpoint is that there are just two opposite answers to every question ("Either outlaw sex in the media or do nothing about it").

The Attorney General's Commission on Pornography, appointed in 1986, attacked the problem with a new mindset. Instead of looking at the early studies exposing a subject only once to the sexual materials, researchers looked at attitudes that changed after watching the media. Researchers were now able to measure sexual arousal to violent material in the laboratory. The idea that people's attitudes can be hurt, even if they don't commit the acts they have seen in the media, was new.

We still did nothing when the 1986 Commission concluded that " . . . substantial exposure to sexually violent materials is a causative factor in antisocial acts of sexual violence."[3] These findings echoed a number of other calls for changes in the media. Studies by the National Institute of Mental Health, the American Psychological Association, and the American Medical Association have concluded that there is overwhelming evidence of television's ability to cause aggressive and violent behavior.[4] The American Academy of Pediatrics has also found that " . . . protracted television viewing is one cause of violent or aggressive behavior."[5] But still, when I present this material in class, many students become as defensive as if I had attacked a close relative.

How do the media actually influence sexual attitudes and behavior? We'll look at these influences separately so we can isolate the influences of sex and violence.

The Humor-Aggression Connection

Do you think it has an effect when millions of Americans, every evening, watch people insulting each other as a primary form of entertainment? (If you don't think this is happening, check off the number of insults between men and women in situation comedies.) On our TV, we actually have comedy shows based entirely on dates insulting one another; or on married people revealing personal and derogatory information—all accompanied by uproarious laughter. Does this constant emphasis on verbal aggression influence our children's views of sexual relationships? Of faithfulness, loyalty, and respect? I think so. There is documented evidence that children often imitate insults they hear in the media.

When hurting someone is portrayed as funny and a laugh track follows, it is virtually impossible for the emotional impact to hit the viewer. It is true that, historically, our entertainment has included aggressive acts, in Punch and Judy shows, the circus, and even cartoons in which the cat smashes the mouse against the wall. But research shows that the more frequently we see aggression, the more realistic and human it is, and the more the aggressor wins, the more it tends to be accepted as natural and the more it is imitated.

One of the most common combinations on TV is sexual aggression with laugh tracks. In situation comedies women insult men's potency or intelligence, and men call women such names as slut and bimbo. Casual, risky sex in a bar scene brings howls of laughter. Watching this type of behavior causes slight attitude shifts over time and allows us to accept things that we would previously have found shocking.

Listen to a randomly chosen episode of a situation comedy, *Married With Children*, that has been rated among the ten most popular programs with Americans eighteen to twenty-five years old:[6]

The teenage sister wiggles her body—dressed in hooker clothes as her younger brother informs her that the Gutter Cats are looking for a dancer. (Taped laughter.)

Sister: "Oh, the Gutter Cats! If I could pick one group to have my baby by, it would be them!" (Taped laughter.)

At the end we see that the group has chained her to a fence; she is wiggling to the music and loving it. (Taped laughter.)

The father comes to "save" her (taped laughter) but he gets distracted by an offer to be in show business.

Sister: "Dad! Untie me!" (Taped laughter.)

Dad: "Shut up!" (Taped laughter.)

Sister: "This is the second time this week someone has chained me to a fence!" (Hilarious laughter.)

In twenty minutes this program enables the viewer to laugh at seductive clothes on a young teen, sexual promiscuity, unwed motherhood, group sex, male domination and bondage, the insensitivity of males who desert a female family member for their own selfish reasons, and a daughter with a self-concept so low that she allows herself to be chained to a fence not once but twice. Yet the lines in this show were so cleverly written that the emotional significance of this exploitation passed by completely without the viewer's awareness. *It was funny.*

Desensitization

Research shows a fascinating tendency of humans to react less and less after repeated exposure to aggression or other shocking experiences. I remember when this experience happened to me, within one hour. Attending a bullfight in Madrid, I saw the big, beautiful animal, trapped in the bullring, look up with sudden shock and bewilderment at the moment when the matador stabbed him in the neck. As he fell dead, the crowd cheered. Even though I had known I was going to a bullfight, I had not integrated the fact that I would see an animal killed for recreation. I was shocked to see these humans slowly trick the bull into coming close enough to stab it to death. I felt tears running down my cheeks. Picadors brought the second bull into the ring. As they killed him, the spectacle brought tears to my eyes, but they did not run down my cheeks. By the time they killed the third bull, I was watching without crying, feeling more detached from the plight of the bull. I observed a number of tourists around me reacting the same way.

Since that day I have never seen an animal killed for entertainment, so I am once again sensitized. But every day we can watch people being hurt. One of my male students commented on his desensitization to a typical "adventure" program on television. In his analysis he wrote: "This program has shown rape, violence, and use of guns to kill people. I was not shocked in the least. None of it appalled me, and I had seen each act of violence before."

Desensitization is not always bad. It enables a surgeon to cut a human body and a mortician to work with the dead. But research shows very clearly that watching television and seeing films desensitizes us to whatever commonly occurs in the programs. We come to accept without a twinge things that, if we saw them for the first time, would inspire anger, sadness, fear, or shock. People from nonviolent societies would flinch and their hearts would pound if they watched the stabbings, shootings, and other murders we can see every day in our own living rooms. Content analyses of the mass media show that by the age of eighteen, the average American has seen 250,000 acts of violence and 40,000 murders or attempted murders on TV.[7] It is not unusual for analyses of program violence on major networks to show forty acts of violence per hour.[8]

The same desensitization results from repeatedly watching sexual exploitation in the media. We stop responding so much to the near-rapes and insults, and the jokes and the teasing become a part of every American's commonplace experience. Where the word *bitch* was once shocking, even a rape attempt can now be accepted with composure.

The media contribute to this callous and insensitive attitude. Do you still have normal sensitivity to violence in the media? Fright or revulsion after seeing media violence is a normal response. **If you do not feel fright or revulsion, you have been desensitized. If you actually enjoy violence, you have experienced serious harmful effects, even if you are not aware of it.**

Watching Sex without Aggression

Earl, eighteen, reads a book called the *Kama Sutra*, an ancient East Indian sex manual with graphic descriptions of consenting sex between adults. He gets aroused while he's reading. Are there any negative effects from this material?

Marty, thirty-one, is powerfully attracted to magazines that show sexual violence. Pictures of men scaring women turn him on. He loves to see a scene of rape portrayed as if the woman enjoyed it. Are there any negative effects from Marty's reading?

The erotic sex that Earl saw and the aggressive sex that turns Marty on are not the same thing. Those who have tried to outlaw what is obscene have not even been able to agree on a definition. But sexually aggressive material is easier to define, since it involves more observable phenomena than does obscenity. Aggression refers to behavior intended to harm someone or something. Earl's book does not involve hurting anyone. Marty's magazine glorifies aggression. Although it may seem that most of the aggression and violence in our country have little influence on our sexual behavior, nothing could be further from the truth.

My students are amazed at the amount of insulting and name-calling in their favorite programs when they are required to analyze them.

Some common examples of aggression are:

Sarcasm
Yelling
Insulting
Name-calling
Vicious gossip
Manipulating by lying
Pushing
Slapping
Hitting, tying up, bruising
Shooting or stabbing, mutilating, hanging, drowning someone.

Most sitcoms and many films depend on the verbal aggression from the first part of the list. But you can see that as aggression intensifies it involves physical actions, which we call violence. In completing the TV analysis at the end of this chapter, my students submit long lists of creative ways to murder people. Such is the way we amuse ourselves by watching the pain and the wounding of our own kind.

Linking sex with aggression is a dangerous way to entertain people. I once heard a psychiatrist request that when Hollywood shows a woman being hurt, they move the aggression at least five minutes from the sexy part so that link will not be so strong. Aggressive acts are often combined in the most fascinating ways with sex, to give the viewer the biggest thrills: A killer bursts in on a woman who is showering; an older man imposes sex upon a young woman who begins by saying no and then loves it; or maybe a couple are just insulting each other—that's aggression between the genders.

Sex is a powerful drive, and most cultures portray sexual satisfaction and delight in visual arts or in literature. Although you may be shocked to see private erotic acts, your astonishment does not mean that they are all harmful; we must be clear on the difference between the merely erotic image and the degrading, aggressive, or violent one.

Those who oppose aggressive sex in the media do not necessarily oppose all sexual content. It is certainly *possible* to make erotic films that are totally nonviolent, which depict a woman as an adult with her own preferences, not as an ever-willing nymphomaniac. Women Against Pornography, an action group opposed both to pornography and censorship, contends that *it is extremely difficult to find portrayals of consenting, mutual, explicit sex between individuals in a caring relationship in the United States.* But even if we could find truly erotic, nondegrading sex where people were really making love, would that be okay for children and teens?

A frequent diet of erotic sexual material may cause sex to seem *unrealistically important,* or stimulate some young people into acts they are better off avoiding. Suppose fifteen-year-old David and his friends watch one of his parents' explicit sexual films one afternoon when they're alone in the house. The next day David goes out with Nancy. They kiss and become very aroused. Mentally, David now has some concrete ideas of what they could be doing. Somehow it's more difficult to believe Nancy's protests. He finds that he's irritated with her. That videotape was so arousing that its images remain. In a way, David feels that Nancy is depriving him, because those women on the tape were so willing, so excited.

Our young people believe "everyone is doing it." If they become prematurely involved in sex, it can be more difficult for them to concentrate on studies and social activities. Erotic or other adult sexual material may also *sexualize children before puberty, making them acutely aware of sexual matters.* Some teachers are noticing increased interest in sex at earlier ages. One middle-school teacher tells me that she frequently intercepts notes from eleven- or twelve-year-old girls. A common message is, "Would you let a boy f - - - you?"

Our culture keeps sex in the forefront of everyone's mind. We now have preteens who dress in a sexually alluring manner, complete with makeup and tight clothes, becoming sexually active. We have twelve-year-olds who are pregnant or infected with STDs. When society promises that sex is the ticket to adulthood, imitation follows. On the other hand, some professionals think that, for adults, *erotica may be a harmless sexual outlet.* It may also be viewed as a positive influence. Sex therapists sometimes advise their clients to read erotic material to help them become aroused. In order to get truly nondegrading erotic video material in our country, however, some therapists must write their own. Explicit erotic material should be restricted to adults. And that means unavailable to children. It is destructive and hypocritical to preach to young teenagers that they are too young to have sex and then pique their interest by portraying sexual themes all around them. It is, at least, good manners to refrain from enticing someone with what he is struggling to avoid. And it clearly is foolhardy to depend upon parents to censor their children's viewing. At least half of parents don't supervise their children's viewing. Surveys indicate that a large percentage of young teenage boys have seen erotic videos and slashers—R-rated films that show extreme violence to women.

The New Media Nymphomaniacs

A rapist was interviewed in prison. He had brutally beaten his victim during the rape. "She liked it rough," he still maintains. It is quite common for a rapist to insist that his victim really enjoyed his attack; he may totally distort her reaction. There are documented cases of both stranger and acquaintance rapists who adamantly contend, sometimes even *during* the rape, that "She loved it."

Social scientists have studied this issue. Pornography showing sex between consenting adults, neither of whom is being dominated or harmed, is known as erotica. There are countless examples in art throughout history. An important modern twist, however, is in the nonviolent erotica that portrays women acting like nymphomaniacs. In *Pornography: Women, Violence, and Civil Liberties*, Corinne Sweet describes the pornography to which boys are now being exposed:[9]

> *Its crude and simplistic messages encourage men to "do it" to women, imply that women are "desperate for it," and that women are smilingly "available," always inviting them sexually, even when they say "no."*

In these films, women are uncontrollably enthusiastic over any sexual suggestion or action from men: screaming for sex, acting ecstatic about any sexual request, no matter how unusual. Solid research suggests that watching a steady diet of this nymphomaniac type of sex, even though it is nonviolent, can be harmful.

Studies at the University of Evansville and Indiana University show that men who watched only one hour of "nympho" films every week for six weeks were more callous toward women. The authors reported that the men were much more accepting of such statements as "A man should find them, feel them, f - - - them, and forget them," or "If they're old enough to bleed, they're old enough to butcher."[10] Remember, these explicit sexual films depict no aggression, but their women characters are so turned on that they can hardly stand it and are begging for more. A number of studies have shown that nymphomaniac pornography causes many normal men to believe that women are more promiscuous than they really are, that women are always ready to be turned on.[11] Quite naturally curious about women and sex, inexperienced young males have few other sources of information about what sex with a women is really like. They can't get the truth in the locker room and they look to the media. Pornography with the insatiable woman, our most common theme, is there to teach them false expectations and a sense of entitlement to the body of a woman with no preferences but theirs.

Watching Aggression Without Sex

Even without sex, violence in the media has a powerful impact on women. Violent films with no sexual content whatsoever cause more aggression against women than films that are *explicitly sexual with no violence*. That is, nonviolent films that contain a lot of sex may be *less* damaging than very violent films with no explicit sex.

Researchers at the University of Wisconsin found disturbing effects in men who had seen just slasher movies, films showing severe violence such as mutilation of women, but with no explicit sex. The male subjects were above average in mental health, since severely disturbed men were excluded. After watching such films as *Texas Chainsaw Massacre* and *Toolbox Murders*, the men's emotional reactions to other filmed violence toward women was dulled. On the last day of the experiment, they rated the level of violence lower than on the first day, even though the slashers were arranged in a different order for different men. By the last day they were so desensitized that they considered the films much less degrading and offensive to women than they had at the beginning. After seeing only three hours of the movies, the men viewed a rape trial they believed to be the real thing from a law school documentary. When asked how hurt the rape victim was, they underestimated the harm to her. They evaluated her as less worthy than did a group who had seen no violence beforehand. They judged the victim to be more responsible for her own sexual assault and felt less sympathy for her on the final day of the viewings.[12] Other researchers have also found that men, especially, recommend a lower prison sentence for a rapist even three weeks after viewing common, nonviolent pornography (explicit sexual portrayals).[13] Even women in the experiment exhibited some of the same changes, but to a lesser degree than those of men.

Rape and fighting are both physical assaults. No society that encourages violence can keep its people sexually safe; the mind of an angry, assaultive person knows no such boundaries. It is impossible to glorify violence to *entertain* people and separate this nonsexual assault from *sexual* assault. Remember Sanday's study of societies with no rape?[14] These societies do not glorify violence in any form, nor do they use it to entertain themselves.

We must confront the facts: *Showing male heroes successfully assaulting other people—whether in films, television, boxing, or football—is the primary form of entertainment in our country.* Female movie stars, who once had at least half of the feature film roles, now complain that they have less than a third.[15] The film industry aims at a target audience of males between sixteen and twenty-five, and this onslaught of macho violence has begun to overwhelm the public with vicious and brutal images and solutions.

Merely protecting the young from nudity and explicit sex acts in the media is too simple. If we try to get rid of only explicit, erotic sex, we ignore the R-rated violence that is the most risky even to adults. Violence against females is committed twice as often in R-rated than in X-rated videos.[16] Avoiding X ratings by substituting a new scale still does not tell the viewer what the film *contains*. If these films are not explicitly sexual, they are usually not X-rated.

Rarely does the American audience learn that most vital message for successful marriage, parenting, and friendship: Conflicts can be resolved without hurting someone. Is it any wonder, then, that every fifteen seconds in this country another woman is beaten up by a man? The message is, when angry, hurt someone.

The Catastrophic Linking of Sex and Aggression

One of my students wrote, "I did see a lot of violence when you gave me this assignment, but then I thought, if there were no violence, TV would be so *boring!*" Many young people believe there's no fun or adventure possible if we omit glorified aggression and exploitative sex. This tragic view, rather than reflecting the truth, reveals the limited environment of the younger generation.

Human experience includes a wide variety of happy, sensuous, and frightening events. Although violence is a part of some people's lives, it is the media *overemphasis on irrelevant, unfeeling* violence used to excite an audience that seems to be the major problem today. There are plenty of possibilities for hilarious or exciting entertainment without glorified violence. And even great literature depicts incidents of sex and violence only briefly when it is vital to the plot. Hamlet had murderous thoughts, but his impulses were interesting to the audience because they were rare; people in Shakespeare's time did not sit around with an electric box tuned to nightly murders committed by powerful heroes and shown in graphic detail. And how many great pieces of literature or theater offer assaults drawn out in vivid technicolor, showing every knife against the breast and every frightened cry, to tantalize and excite the viewer as the woman tries vainly to escape? It is a recent phenomenon for an audience to see a human being inflict bloody injuries, rape, or death upon another person with such frequency and in such a manner. In the history of American film, there have been scores of fascinating storylines without this kind of emphasis.

Extreme Aggression: Violent Sex

Watching harm to a person who *does not like* being hurt offers at least one kind of reality: The sensitive viewer has a chance to learn that victims *really suffer*. But showing a victim who *likes being victimized* is the most dangerous kind of sexual depiction.

A few years ago I announced to my class, "Next week we will talk about rape." "Hooray!" yelled a young man in the front row, grinning and clapping his hands. Where did he learn to view rape as such great fun?

The National Coalition on Television Violence—which analyzes films and other media—reports that one out of eight Hollywood films depicts a rape.[17] If you watch carefully you will find that some type of sex without consent—even if it's a comic character peeking in on a woman dressing—occurs with astonishing regularity in the movies. These intrusions are woven into the plot, and we may not realize we've seen them, so brainwashed are we. When I asked fifty students who had seen *Pretty Woman* how many of them were aware that there was a rape attempt in the film, *70 percent of the students did not remember the attempted rape*, although a man had thrown a woman on the floor and tried to pull off her clothes. Her boyfriend saved her, nothing bad seemed to result, and so they forgot. Sexual violence is so common that we underreact to it, just as we take for granted the sight of a gun on the screen, a weapon for killing human beings.

A surprising percentage of rape survivors claim that their attackers were either talking about or looking at pornographic material just before or during the assault. Rape survivors are not the only women who have felt the influence of pornography. Sociologist Diana Russell surveyed 930 women for the National Institute of Mental Health. "Have you ever been upset by anyone trying to get you to do what they'd seen in pornographic pictures, movies, or books?" Ten percent of the women answered that they had been upset by such an experience at least once.[18] Researcher W. L. Marshall cites three studies showing that as many as one-third of rapists and child molesters purposely use pornography either during or immediately after their crimes. It is difficult, according to Marshall, to resist the conclusion that pornography has a negative effect on these criminals. Russell makes no apologies for taking a stand against pornography and feels that researchers do not have to bend over backward to be neutral in the face of prevailing evidence.[20] Among the points she documents are these:

1. Testimony from a high percentage of rapists and child molesters quotes them as saying that pornography inspired them to commit crimes. (Ted Bundy is an example who admitted this in his testimony.)

2. Research finds normal, healthy male students saying that, after being exposed once to violent pornography, they are more likely to rape a woman.

3. Studies indicate that large percentages of men ranging from junior high through adulthood report imitating X-rated movies within a few days after seeing them.

4. Hundreds of women have publicly testified that they have been victimized by pornography, often being pressured to engage in actions the men learned about from pornography.

5. Experimental research has shown that viewing violent pornography results in higher rates of aggression against women by male subjects.

We would not entertain ourselves with the sexual torture of any other group but women. Cruelty to animals still repels us because we have not been witnessing its dramatization every night for years. If we did to animals and children what we do to women in the media, there would be such a public outcry that it would be stopped overnight. The same holds true for disrespect to minority groups. No sponsor would dare to put on a program that portrayed any group besides women being tortured and mutilated. But we've slowly been lulled into thinking that the scared woman and the violent man are a natural part of entertainment. In a sense, the media actually train viewers to sexually victimize human beings. They not only train viewers in how personally to victimize people, they prepare viewers to accept it calmly when others victimize people.

Rather than present the hundreds of research findings about sexual influence from the media, let's *summarize* the most prominent findings of recent, university-based research projects:[21] Most of these researchers use the word *pornography* to refer to the sexually explicit material that they study: Pornography can be non-violent (mutual pleasure in lovemaking); degrading (there are insults or physical acts that are demeaning); or violent (somebody is physically hurt or forced during sexual acts).

What If the Sex is Degrading but Nonviolent?

In this kind of porn, a man does something that may be considered demeaning, such as assuming a dominant position over a woman and masturbating into her face—and she is depicted as loving it. Or he dominates her as if she were a child under his control. In summarizing the results of forty-six separate studies by thirty-eight scientists, Zillmann and Bryant report some appalling results in both men and women from prolonged consumption of "common" pornography, that which[22] is most commonly found in our society. Although not violent, the sex is instant, it's between strangers, and the woman is invariably portrayed as a plaything who is eager to be used sexually by the male in any way. Look at the changes in both men and women after watching just six hours of common pornography:

TABLE 9-1   Effects of Prolonged Viewing of Pornography on Normal Subjects

Sexual arousal.	Becoming more tolerant of their partners' having sex with others.
Less and less feeling of revulsion.	Becoming much more tolerant of acts that are "improper" or in bad taste.
Needing more and more unusual porn to become aroused.	Expressing less desire to have children.
Preferring porn that contains less common sexual acts.	Expressing more doubts about the value of marriage.
Believing that unusual sex acts are more popular than they really are.	Becoming less content with their partners' physical appearance.
Becoming more tolerant of the idea of extramarital sex.	Becoming less content with their partners' sexual behavior.
Viewing rape as a more trivial offense.	Believing child abuse is a less serious offense.

When male viewers in some studies had watched pornography that was more violent than our common pornography, they became even less sensitive toward victims of sexual violence. Asked what kind of sexual force they felt capable of, many believed themselves more capable of forcing oral sex or other sexual acts short of rape on a reluctant female. And they believed themselves more capable of committing rape, particularly the more disturbed male subjects. They began to view violence as routine. When put into a situation where they believed they were witnessing a rape, they were less likely to help the victim than nonviewers of pornography. (Fortunately, all subjects were debriefed at the end of experiments to cancel any negative effects.)

What if Aggression is Added to Degrading Pornography?

This kind of porn shows men insulting or even causing pain to women through beatings or other physical acts. They may be called names (often sexual: bitch, slut, whore), slapped, or held at the point of a knife or gun, but end up crazy about the guy. A number of soaps have also shown rape victims falling in love with the men who raped them. These movies go much further than the women-love-all-sex films, which are not aggressive enough to be called violent. The women in the I-love-force films are not always raped, but there is enough aggressive stuff to make it clear that they like it rough. And these films about women who enjoy or are aroused by violence change the attitudes of many men who watch them. In the studies, viewers became more callous and accepting of violence and they believed more of the rape myths such as those on page 139. When a laboratory experiment was set up where they could deliver a punishment of electric shock to a woman or a man, the viewers of violence punished only the woman, and they punished her much more than did men who had seen a purely erotic film.[23] (In reality, no electric shock was delivered.) Whether a male becomes aggressive after viewing pornography depends on a number of factors. But researchers at the University of California at Santa Barbara believe there is great risk to adolescent males who have access to this kind of media violence.

If pornography damages normal men, what are its effects on rapists? Only about one in 15,000 rapists is convicted. And one in twelve American males admits to acts that meet the legal definition of rape.[24] Since our experts estimate that 25 percent of American females are raped, we must conclude that thousands of rapists are free and unpunished in our society. They are often repeaters. When a woman is raped on a TV show, nudity is not shown. But even rape images that do not show nudity can have dangerous effects on rapists. Researchers have found that rapists become aroused by seeing images of a man being aggressive toward a woman, even omitting sex. Such behaviors as pushing, shoving, slapping, insulting, or otherwise hurting a woman are a real turn-on.

The Problem with Macho

In 1993 a man killed his son because he was playing with dolls. The father was afraid his son was going to become a homosexual. What we define as masculine invites many sexual tragedies. We should be deeply concerned that the macho male, the insensitive guy who loves violence, is so much admired. To the macho man, the world is divided into tough guys and wimps, and relationships are risky because he will lose the total control that props up his sense of masculinity. Some researchers at the University of Connecticut have proposed a "macho personality" with the following characteristics:[25]

- Callous sex attitudes toward women
- Celebration of male aggressiveness
- Fascination with danger

Psychotherapists are in agreement that we create an emotional vacuum in young men by squelching all emotions but anger. We instruct little boys not to cry, although it's a human, and not exclusively female, reaction. We somehow imply that tenderness is feminine. We encourage men to be constantly courageous and show no fear. All of these pressures can produce men *who cannot feel*. Those who score high on tests of macho attitudes show this lack of sensitivity. They express no interest in a raped woman's well-being; they see her as just an object on which to score.[26] If we socialize men to believe that the greatest achievements in life are power, domination, toughness, strength, aggressiveness, and the ability to compete, how can we expect them not to carry these values into the area of sex? Millions of young Americans do not even know that masculinity can be defined any other way. In 1993 rape charges against members of the Spur Posse, a group of young teens who gave points for sex with the most females, showed how easily macho can get out of hand. In their frenzy to put more notches on their belts, they were accused of sexual assault and rape, and one of the victims was ten years old. But the boys' fathers were not ashamed; a number of them couldn't understand all the fuss and accused the girls of being sluts. Some researchers believe that "macho" makes men more afraid of *each other* than of anything else; being a wimp is the most dreaded thing of all.[27]

Myriam Miedzian, in her book *Boys Will Be Boys*, makes a compelling case for teaching our sons a new kind of masculinity that will result in peaceful men with a more mature courage:[28]

> . . . *There are many gentle, sensitive, caring men in this world, and they are not "wimps," as popular prejudice would have it. Their sensitivity is often joined with unusual courage, curiosity, sense of adventure, and independence from societal pressures. . . . These are the kinds of men I*

know, admire, and find attractive. . . . I have been able to see that men do not have to be the victims of dysfunctional, destructive, atavistic male archetypes. . . .

A young adolescent male is anxious to learn how to treat a woman. He's not going to learn any healthy ways from macho men. At one time, older adolescents indoctrinated younger males to the world of sex in the bull session; now the pornography and sexual violence that young teenagers consume is their "primary sexual indoctrination."[29]

Females Who Encourage Macho in Men

Many women are fascinated with the rascal, the rough guy who is difficult (if they only knew, impossible) to get. He's impossible because he can't form a close intimate relationship. I've heard male students complain that nice guys finish last. I can tell that these men feel pressure to act macho because they rarely say anything sensitive in class but often do so alone in my office. I tell them, nice guys will not finish last. But if you love a woman who wants you to be a little meaner, a little rougher, with her, she couldn't have a healthy relationship with you anyway. Be yourself, and if she won't change and appreciate you, move on.

Is a sensitive man a turnoff? One experiment showed that young women who watched slashers with men found the men *who did not react* to the violence more attractive than those who appeared distressed by all the blood and brutality.[30] Has a "real man" come to mean one who can watch victimization without feelings? Some women may subtly reward men for the very kinds of attitudes that could result in their own victimization. This does not mean they are to blame, because the perpetrator of a crime is responsible for restraining himself. An assertive woman does not usually find herself in this situation, nor is she usually chosen by a macho male. Self-confidence in a woman is a threat and a turnoff to a macho male. Equality scares him because he cannot be the only powerful one in such a relationship.

We have provided a superb training ground for sexual violence. If a Martian arrived on earth and asked for assistance in helping him learn calmly to degrade, torture, rape, or mutilate human beings, we would know exactly how to teach it. Our entertainment has made us experts.

Facing the Truth

But is laboratory research really a reflection of life? Laboratory experiments on pornography are so carefully controlled that, if anything, they are thought to underestimate the effect of pornography on the subject's aggressive responses. Some studies even eliminated highly disturbed males from their groups and still found the viewers of violence more willing to hurt a woman. The advantage of a controlled laboratory *experiment* is that the *causes* of human behavior can be demonstrated. The experiment is a powerful device for finding clear causes, which is why we respect the experimental method so much in medical research.

These findings are based upon summaries of numerous careful research studies. The major researchers in the field are convinced enough of the harm of aggression in the media to devote their careers to exploring this problem. Scientists are engaged in additional research to examine further the complex connections between sex and violence.

Why do we ignore these findings? If many medical studies revealed, say, that a steady consumption of apples harmed large numbers of people, if the bulk of scientific studies showed that apple consumption created a health risk, apples would certainly bear warning labels at the very least. Only the apple growers' lobby would argue, "Not everyone is hurt by apples. You can't prove apples hurt people. Don't put warning labels on them!" When a drug is suspected of causing cancer in rats, let alone humans, it is usually withdrawn. Part of the problem is that, short of censorship, we have not known what to do. In so many ways, Americans sit helplessly and watch the social fabric of their country deteriorate.

Strong feelings have grown up about our rights to sexual material. There is an incredible ignorance of the research that I've cited. Some people try to portray moderate, concerned citizens as threats to freedom. All of us who stand up on this issue must be prepared for criticism; but living in fear of sexual exploitation is certainly a threat to freedom. We have a right to go about our lives freely without the restrictions necessary to avoid sex offenders. We must have the courage to insist that we be heard. We must welcome the debate over this issue, no matter how heated it becomes. We must have a clear understanding of censorship issues. *Protesting the kinds of media that cause documented harm is very different from trying to censor art forms from which no harm has ever been demonstrated.* Trying to eliminate sex from all forms of artistic expression is an uninformed and oppressive action. But ignoring research about what is detrimental to our society is courting disaster.

When Is it Okay to Portray Sex or Violence?

If most young people saw strong caring relationships in their families, perhaps they could emerge from years of this media barrage without damage. But millions of young Americans have never seen a man and woman treat each other with caring and respect, much less lived with a married couple in harmony. They are especially defenseless against the hours of sick images they watch on TV. We need to depict healthy relationships in exciting, adventurous stories. We can make aggressive sex in the media shocking and in bad taste, just as we have done with racism. We can make it unfashionable and unprofitable to portray these views in the media. After all, smoking in certain public places is now taboo, but thirty years ago it was taken for granted. Attitude changes are possible.

Although there is some evidence that prolonged exposure to erotic sex might change what men expect of women, media sex between consenting adults is certainly healthier fare than exploitative or violent sex. We can even portray violence alone if it is not glorified and if it is realistic. If a story involves someone's being hurt—in war, rape, or even through milder aggression—*let the camera or the book show the real pain and hurt of that person.* The National Coalition on Television Violence *recommends* certain realistic war films, because they do not glorify violence. In genuine sexual relationships, adult women dislike force and men reject force as a way of loving.

We must look for alternatives to censorship. If scientists continue to prove that our media portray sex in a manner constituting a clear and present danger, then further debate on censorship will no doubt occur. But we can also take actions that are alternatives to censorship.

Rating Your Favorite Movies and TV Programs

How many destructive sexual messages occur in your favorite programs or films? Sexual exploitation is influenced by sexual and nonsexual violence. Use the first checklist below to rate sexual messages and the second to rate the violent messages in general. Test yourself for desensitization; if you are surprised at your total scores, you have been desensitized.

Sexual Messages in the Media

During a single program or film, or while looking at a magazine, check any of the following that occur (ignore whether there is laughter):

__ 1. Characters show hostility by calling names or insulting the opposite sex.

__ 2. Characters manipulate and play games in love relationships; that is, they are deceptive:

    __ they lie to their spouses about sex
    __ they lie to get sex from someone
    __ they otherwise deceive a sex partner

__ 3. One gender dominates the other (use of power).

__ 4. Jokes or put-downs about commitment (such as jokes about how bad marriage is).

__ 5. Couple has intercourse without mention of birth control.

__ 6. Couple has intercourse occurring without mention of disease risk.

__ 7. Men or women make uninvited remarks about the secondary sex characteristics (breasts, etc.) of another person.

__ 8. Characters have titillating attitude about sex (making sexual implications out of events that are really not sexual) or they giggle about double meanings of words that could be interpreted as sexual.

__ 9. Men or women publicly put down the sexual abilities of another person.

__10. Character laughs at serious sexual problems (comedies that joke about unwed parenthood, deception, disease, prostitution, etc.).

__11. Women or men are consistently portrayed as stupid.

__12. An employer or fellow employee makes sexual remarks to another employee, or engages in more serious sexual harassment.

__13. Characters engage in sexual aggression or violence irrelevant to the plot (ranging from insults to rape).

__14. Males are portrayed as insensitive.

__15. Males are portrayed as more interested in sexual conquests than in the woman's feelings.

__16. Women are portrayed as weak or frightened.

__17. Women are portrayed as not really minding sexual force, or as liking it.

__18. Rape is attempted (regardless of whether victim began to like it).

__19. A completed rape is shown.

__20. Program or film implies rape myths:

    __ women are always interested in sex
    __ men cannot help but be sex-driven
    __ other rape myths (list on p. 139):

__21. Other forms of sexual aggression or exploitation:

Aggressive Incidents in the Media

During a single program or film *make tally marks* to keep a record of each time any of the following occur (ignore whether there is laughter):

VERBAL AGGRESSION (people say things aimed at hurting someone):

__ sarcasm (characters show anger through their tone of voice).

__ threats (about psychological or physical harm that one character may carry out).

__ screaming or yelling at another person, rather than talking to him respectfully.

__ making remarks that degrade or put down another person or group.

__ telling untrue and destructive things behind a person's back.

__ frightening someone anonymously (such as over the telephone).

__ other verbal aggression:

NONVERBAL (PHYSICAL) AGGRESSION:

__ smashing or destroying objects.

__ pushing or shoving.

__ shooting with a weapon.

__ poisoning.

__ stabbing.

__ war (justified, approved aggression.) Describe how the people were hurt:

__ using a car to hurt a person.

__ miscellaneous aggression: drowning, strangling, tripping, pushing off cliff, etc. Describe:

OTHER PHYSICAL AGGRESSION:

Did the media present this violence realistically and sensitively, indicating that it harmed a human being?__ Or was it presented in a glorified way, irrelevant to the storyline, or less serious and tragic than it warranted?__ Do you feel that you reacted the same way to the violence you saw as you would have seeing it on the screen for the first time?__ After writing this checklist, did you become any more aware of anything about aggression and violence in the media? If so, what?

Notes

1. Margaret Mead, "A Proposal: We Need Taboos on Sex at Work," *Redbook* no. 6 (April 1978), 31, 33, 38.

2. Sandra Campbell, "Creating Redemptive Imagery," in Buchwald, Fletcher, and Roth, eds., *Transforming a Rape Culture*, 149.

3. *Attorney General's Commission on Pornography, Final Report* (Washington, D.C.: U.S. Department of Justice, July 1986), 324–26.

4. As discussed in Edward Donnerstein, Daniel Linz, and Steven Penrod, *The Question of Pornography* (New York: The Free Press, 1987), 118; *St. Louis Post-Dispatch* 26 February 1992, A2.

5. Thomas E. Radecki, ed., *NCTV News* 11, no. 3–5. (April–June, 1990), 14.

6. *Married With Children* episode shown at 8 P.M. Sunday, July 22, 1990. Channel 30, St. Louis, Missouri.

7. Daniel Linz, Barbara J. Wilson, and Edward Donnerstein, "Sexual Violence in the Mass Media: Legal Solutions, Warnings, and Mitigation Through Education," *Journal of Social Issues* 48, no. 1 (1992): 146.

8. Radecki, *NCTV News*, 9.

9. Corinne Sweet, "Pornography and Addiction: A Political Issue," in Catherine Itzin, ed., *Pornography: Women, Violence, and Civil Liberties* (New York: Oxford University Press, 1992), 179–80.

10. Dolf Zillmann and Jennings Bryant, "Effects of Massive Exposure to Pornography," in Donnerstein, Linz, and Penrod, eds., *Pornography and Sexual Aggression* (New York: Academic Press, 1984), 115–38.

11. Dolf Zillmann and James B. Weaver, "Pornography and Men's Sexual Callousness toward Women," in Dolf Zillman and Jennings Bryant, eds., *Pornography: Research Advances and Policy Considerations*, (Hillsdale, N.J., 1989), 95–125.

12. Daniel Linz, "Sexual Violence in the Media: Effects on Male Viewers and Implications for Society" (unpublished doctoral dissertation, University of Wisconsin, 1985); Daniel Linz, Edward Donnerstein, and Steven Penrod, "The Effects of Multiple Exposures of Filmed Violence Against Women," *Journal of Communication* 34 (1984): 130.

13. Dolf Zillmann, "Effects of Prolonged Consumption of Pornography," in Zillmann and Bryant, eds., *Pornography: Research Advances and Policy Considerations*, 127–57.

14. Sanday, "Socio-Cultural Context of Rape."

15. "Women Lament Loss of Roles," *St. Louis Post-Dispatch*, 10 August, 1990.

16. Ni Yang and Daniel Linz, "Movie Ratings and the Content of Adult Videos:

The Sex-Violence Ratio," *Journal of Communication* 40, no. 2 (Spring 1990): 28.

17. As reported in *Newsweek* 16 July 1990, 24.

18. Diana E. H. Russell, *Sexual Exploitation* (Newbury Park, Calif.: Sage Library of Social Research, 1984), 124.

19. W. L. Marshall, "Pornography and Sex Offenders," in Zillmann and Bryant, eds., *Pornography: Research Advances and Policy Considerations*, 185–214.

20. Diana E. H. Russell, "Pornography and Rape: A Causal Model," in Catherine Itzin, ed., *Pornography: Women, Violence, and Civil Liberties* (New York: Oxford University Press, 1992), 346.

21. Malamuth and Donnerstein, eds., *Pornography and Sexual Aggression*; Donnerstein, Linz, and Penrod, *The Question of Pornography*; Zillmann and Bryant, eds., *Pornography: Research Advances.*

22. Dolf Zillmann, "Effects of Prolonged Consumption of Pornography," in Zillmann and Bryant, eds., *Pornography: Research Advances*, 153–55. This paper is an updated version of a paper commissioned by the Surgeon General for the Surgeon General's Workshop on Pornography and Public Health, 1986.

23. Donnerstein, Linz, and Penrod, eds., *The Question of Pornography*, 158.

24. Warshaw, *I Never Called it Rape.*

25. D. L. Mosher and M. Sirkin, "Measuring a Macho Personality Constellation," *Journal of Research in Personality* 18 (1984): 150.

26. As reported in Dolf Zillmann and James B. Weaver, "Pornography and Men's Sexual Callousness Toward Women," Zillmann and Bryant, eds., *Pornography: Research Advances*, 102.

27. Michael S. Kimmel, "Clarence, William, Iron Mike, Tailhook, Senator Packwood, Spur Posse, Magic . . . and Us," in Buchwald, Fletcher, and Roth, eds., *Transforming a Rape Culture*, 19.

28. Myriam Miedzian, *Boys Will Be Boys.*

(New York: Anchor Books, 1991), xxi.

29. As reported in Zillmann and Weaver, "Pornography and Men's Sexual Callousness Toward Women," Zillmann and Bryant, eds., *Pornography: Research Advances*, 102.

30. Dolf Zillmann et. al., "Effects of the Opposite-Gender Companion's Affect to Horror or Distress, Delight and Attraction," *Journal of Personality and Social Psychology* 51 (1986): 586.

10

Becoming a Witness

Which side are you on?[1]
—PROTEST SONG BY FLORENCE REECE
HARLAN COUNTY, KENTUCKY

How will you speak, how will you use your strength and come out of your silence and stand up for justice? For it is not enough to assert yourself just for your personal welfare. You have a lot to gain if those around you are safe from sexual exploitation and abuse. Trying to ensure only your *own* safety in a sick society is like taking an antibiotic when an infection is rampant in your community; it may come back to you if it is not stamped out. You will pay for all the social services required to cope with these misfortunes. Your money will pay for police, health costs, therapists, prisons, and even for many of the children of teenage mothers. But most important, you will be trying to exist in a country where every fourth or fifth person is a survivor. Even if you are never victimized, you will discover that your friends, your spouse and children, and the people your children decide to befriend or marry may be among these exploited people, some of whom will still be suffering. The bell tolls for you.

We have seen that you cannot separate what's good for women from what's best for men. When a society allows one to be put down, the other suffers from the lonely struggle to remain unfeeling and dominant. And you cannot separate sexual violence from other kinds of violence, because societies that encourage hurting people will show vicious and brutal solutions even when making "love." If your consciousness has been raised by this book—if you can hardly go to the movies now without being aware of sexual exploitation—that's good. Becoming acutely aware of what we should not tolerate will drive us out of our silence. It is a normal response to feel ashamed or uncomfortable when we sit calmly in the face of insults to our humanity. Humans are capable of living together without hurting each other, and there is no satisfaction like that of rising to our potential.

But how can we have an impact? You do not have to be radical or go to a great deal of personal effort to cause social change. It just takes a lot of people who are fed up. Every week there are opportunities for you to show that you have high standards. The most effective ways to turn things around are available to you every day in social and business situations. And if you do decide to engage in organized protest, we Americans have a great tradition of challenging the status quo. Our country was founded on it.

"But," you object, "I don't contribute to any sexual exploitation." Your silence has an immense impact. Your lack of involvement permits the problems I've described to be socially acceptable. To paraphrase Edmund Burke, "The only thing necessary for the triumph of evil is for good people to do nothing." *By your actions, you are a witness to your beliefs.*

There is ample research to demonstrate that other people interpret *silence* as *approval*. A study of junior high gossip by Donna Eders at Indiana University found that it is the comment made after the gossip that is critical.[2] If the listener expressed agreement, the gossip escalated. Once one person seconded a smear against someone, no one ever challenged it. But regardless of how insulting the opening remark was, an immediate disagreement could send the gossip in a less critical direction.[3] I believe these same principles apply to sexist put-downs and rape myths.

Instead of thinking it's about "them" and doesn't concern you, think of exploitative films, jokes, or remarks as attacks on your own family. Because they are. Have the same courage to speak up against these sick influences as you would if your own mother, sister, or brother were being criticized.

Where to Begin

This chapter will show you how to put pressure at three points:

1. How to talk back directly to people around you about unhealthy sexual messages.
2. How to influence the media to use their creative capacities in prosocial—rather than antisocial—ways.
3. How to insist on education at all points where it can have impact.

The clarity of your position will decrease the chances that anyone would dare to offend you by making light of your feelings. Such assertiveness is the reason the media can no longer portray African Americans as eye-rolling cowards or stupid servants. After years of antiracists' hard work and protest, a social stigma results from presenting Blacks in such a negative light. For the same reason, funny drunks no longer show up on television, *because millions of Americans disapprove.* You can learn ways to make your society feel the stubborn ounces of your weight, so that we might tip the scale in favor of sexual justice.

In case you're worried that you can't fit the mold of a social activist, there is still a place for you. There are varying styles of assertiveness. If you think of yourself as a shy person who cannot live up to this powerful assertive image, read on. There are ways you can become mature enough to stand for something. All of us have been shocked speechless by other people's remarks and have kicked ourselves later for failing to speak up. If we practice making our voices heard, we can be prepared for the next time.

How to Speak Up in Social and Business Situations

Opportunities constantly arise to talk back in ordinary social situations: jokes among friends, sexist remarks in the workplace, sexual aggression in movies that you see with a date or with friends, and exploitative advertisements from someone who wants your business.

When You Hear Exploitative Jokes

What you find humorous indicates to others where you draw the line. But I have laughed at a joke before I even realized it was offensive, and, probably, so have you. Increasing our awareness is the answer. Be aware when the skillful telling of a joke makes you laugh at something that really isn't funny. There are many jokes about exhibitionism or obscene phone callers, for example, that contribute to the cultural climate of sick sex. If you think about it you will have the remarkable insight that all those funny jokes are not about something that has happened to you, but about another group. People to whom these offenses have happened don't laugh.

It is easy for the exploitative aspects of a story to go right past us. One of my students heard the following joke: "Why did God invent booze? So that fat girls could have a chance to get laid."

In two sentences this joke manages to degrade obese people, women, men, and religion; it also implies that it's acceptable to use a woman sexually if the man numbs himself with alcohol. And it links irresponsible sex and drugs. No doubt many jokes could be picked apart and found unfair to someone. In the last few years I have heard a number of jokes about AIDS and even one about breast cancer. At a conference I heard a talk by a young college woman, infected with HIV by her boyfriend who had injected steroids in high school. She confided that hearing AIDS jokes made it very difficult for her to be upbeat about her struggle.

This won't make you humorless. I hope you have lots of good laughs; I love jokes (although remembering them is a problem) and I think we need to laugh more, not less. It's good for our health, and we deserve some happiness. Norman Cousins dramatically demonstrated the power of laughter when he showed himself comedy videotapes to make himself well again.[4] There are so many harmless funny things we have not even explored. And jokes can still be about sex. Learn to discriminate between an exploitative or degrading joke and a just-plain-funny joke. Be aware of all the good laughs you can have that are not at somebody else's expense. Especially if you are a woman, some folks may actually accuse you of having no sense of humor. You might point out that no one expects other survivors to laugh at jokes about their pain. Do we expect African Americans to laugh at jokes about slavery or lynchings, or Jews about the Holocaust? Then why should women—or anyone—laugh at jokes about sexual exploitation?

Since laughing at an exploitative joke actively supports the wrong side, you need simple skills to cope with such situations. You could make an I-statement in response to a joke, but if you feel uncomfortable coming on too strong, you could do it in a conversational way:

"Well, jokes about women being pushed . . . just turn me off."

"Why am I not laughing? I guess because . . . jokes about _____ just don't seem funny to me."

"I realize people laugh about flashers, but I know some women who were really scared by one"

"You know, I dislike laughing about men's sexual failures."

We have to admit we are human. For one thing, the clever twist put on jokes can make them funny on the surface. If you realize immediately that you've just laughed at something destructive, you could always say, "I laughed at that, but now that I think about it, that joke makes fun of hurting someone." Remember, there are options for you between rage and silence. If you are seated next to the boss at a dinner party, realistically you may not feel you can risk a total scene. Your body language matters here; a blank stare or stunned silence has some impact.

Former first lady Barbara Bush attended a sixtieth birthday party for a politician from the West. In his remarks he said, "I never thought I'd be sleeping with a sixty-year-old woman!" Barbara Bush is reputed to have given him a cold, "Not funny." Once again, those in power may have no trouble speaking out—but she did it concisely, did she not?

Other ways for you to squelch the offensive remark:

"I don't find that amusing."

" . . . (Name a person who has been through that) probably wouldn't laugh at that one."

"I don't think that's funny."

For a more intense situation, or if you want to escalate your remarks:

"I can't believe you said that. I know people who have been through. . . . "

Other kinds of I-statements can be appropriate:

"I get so mad when I hear jokes like that. Don't you remember when I received all those obscene calls and how scared I was?"

Even to a casual acquaintance you could comment:

"Could we talk about something else? I really feel uncomfortable laughing about this. Some of my friends have been . . . ."

Challenge the Myths

Learn to correct myths easily in your conversations:

A: Yeah, but she was drinking when she went to his room, so what did she expect?
B: Wait a minute! Having a drink is not giving consent to have sex.

(Or): *A:* You could hardly blame a man for getting excited and wanting to keep going.
B: Yes, but getting excited isn't the same as forcing someone—that's a felony.

When You See Movies or Programs With Others

Here is one of your best chances to influence your peers. There's research to back up the idea—and it works. Scientists at the University of California found that what women say, or don't say, about an exploitative movie can have a powerful effect on men.[5] The researchers arranged for men and women to view sexually aggressive films together. The study was designed to see whether the females' comments had any effect on the male's attitudes. In some cases the females were told to make positive or negative comments about the films. In other cases they were instructed to remain silent.

The exciting part of this research is that, when the females were negative or neutral in what they said about the films, the males tended to find the films more embarrassing, upsetting, and degrading to women. The authors say that "the presence of a coviewer may have dramatic effects on a person's reactions to sexual violence in the media. . . . The female coviewer served an 'educational' function when she expressed dislike for the film and when she merely watched the depiction in silence."[6] Once again, *when a woman likes to see violence she may unintentionally send a self-destructive message.*

But these same researchers wondered about the old dilemma—would women be afraid of rejection if they were assertive about the films? In one of the studies the researchers looked at the male's attitudes towards the female after she stated her opinions. The results showed that the males could handle female assertiveness, and the fear of being rejected was not borne out. This research offers perhaps the most powerful advice of any in this book, and it is simple: Miss no opportunity to *tell him what you think about sexual violence.*

What a powerful piece of knowledge! Women—and sensitive men—have in their own voice the ability to change others' distorted attitudes. If all those who understand this issue express their disapproval, think what an impact they can have. A woman who is watching a movie or program containing sexual aggression could make various comments about mild, moderate, or severe aggression:

"I don't like to watch that. The people spend so much time putting each other down."

"It was supposed to be a joke, but when they were all laughing about her body, I felt very uncomfortable."

"I resent it when hurting a woman is a form of entertainment. I think it's sick."

"Have you ever noticed how they always put in something sexual where the woman says no but then she likes it? I hate to see that in a movie. Nobody likes to be treated that way."

"Did you notice the attempted rape in that movie? It's getting to be so common we hardly notice." (or): "I can't watch this. I don't like to see people being hurt this way. I'd like to leave."

But I Can't Talk Like That

If you're afraid to speak up around your friends, practice taking small risks. You don't have to make a speech from a soapbox. "Come on, guys, I don't like to see people treated like that. Let's watch something else."

If you're reluctant to speak up to people who watch movies or programs with you, just think about what that means. You have to walk on eggshells and not defend your own healthy beliefs for fear of someone else's disapproval. Any person who would reject you for speaking up about these things is already brainwashed. If you like a man who resents your dislike of violence, your chances of a good relationship with such a man are very slim, if they exist at all. Many men are capable of sensitivity to sexual aggression—if only they have experiences that sensitize, rather than desensitize, them.

Although our view of men needs changing, taking women out of the victim role is most critical. In *Transforming a Rape Culture*, I have described three groups of men with respect to this issue:

There are hard-core, completely macho, insensitive, and callous males. Nothing will change them; their personalities are probably so insecure that they need to control women. At the other extreme are sensitive males who decry the rape culture and don't need their consciousness raised. But in between there are millions of males who are not emotionally invested in misogyny [woman-hating]—they just go along with it. These men in the middle need to be set straight. There is much hope for them. They need to be reminded that the cultural messages are inaccurate. They need to hear someone say, "I don't like jokes that put women down." They need to have peers, friends, teachers, and sisters who speak up when they are hurt, scared, or offended. Otherwise this culture will brainwash men with such overwhelming frequency that they will have no reason to think anyone disapproves.[7]

Other Chances to Respond

What should you say when a business or company displays something sexually degrading or exploitative? Suppose you see an offensive ad or picture on a product's packaging. There are assertive ways to convey your disapproval to the business involved. One young woman wrote a letter to a clothing company:

I thought you might like to have some feedback about your advertising. It really disturbs me to see a young woman in an extremely sexy pose, hitchhiking on a deserted road wearing the clothes you're trying to sell. I won't buy from someone whose advertisements suggest trying to get sex from a pick-up.

Sarah Ciriello, editor of the *Challenging Media Images of Women Newsletter,* suggests these guidelines for letters:[8]

1. Tell them who you are.

2. Describe the product or image that offended you and include a copy if possible.

3. Use statistics if available to strengthen your argument.

4. Ask that the company reconsider its ad or product to become more socially responsible.

5. Mention that you will boycott if necessary.

6. Suggest positive alternatives for the company.

7. Specify target groups to whom you are sending copies of your letter, such as newspaper and TV editors and reporters, state and local organizations.

Insist on Fairness to Men

It's easy to become furious over the wrongs done to women. But consider the number of men who are locked in silence, unable to feel any emotion but anger. There are thousands of divorces where the woman complained that she wanted more sensitivity but the man was not socialized that way. Wherever our consciousness needs to be raised about women, there are myths about men. We need to be consistent and extend our disapproval to destructive images of men:

"Come on, Jill, I really get irritated when you make men sound like they have no self-control."

"Don't make fun of a man crying. We're human, too."

Make Phone Calls

You can make a complaint even to out-of-town companies, often by looking up their 800 numbers. Several groups have caused ads to be canceled when sexist issues were pointed out to the companies. For example, a pharmacy canceled a Valentine's Day radio ad in which a man with an accent obviously imitating Arnold Schwarzenegger recited,

> *Roses are red, violets are blue*
> *You'd better be my valentine,*
> *or I'll pump you full of lead*
> *or I'll shoot you in the head . . .*
> *or you're better off dead.*[9]

How to Refer Someone for Help

When you hear someone who has sexual, drug, or other problems and doesn't know where to turn, consider referring that individual for help. You don't have to be a professional to know where people can get help for alcohol abuse, drug problems or other kinds of personal problems (See Appendix). If the person has asked you for help, you could offer information: "I've heard of a place where you can find out about that. I'll look it up for you if you want me to."

If it's a family member or someone else you love, you can just start with an I-statement and take it from there: "I've been worried about you. I've noticed you seem to feel so bad, and I want us to get you some help with this."

What if the person seems desperate, but doesn't ask you for help? You could still bring up the subject: "You know something, John?, I've heard you talk so many times about how much this upsets you. Did you know there's an agency that helps people with that kind of problem? I have the phone number if you want it."

Speaking Up to the Media

Get everyone you can to phone station executives to complain about ads or programs you find offensive. Already, protest groups have persuaded the media to keep a number of violent programs off the air.

Boycott All Products that Involve Sexual Exploitation

Why buy *any* product that encourages unhealthy sexual attitudes? You may have to stop reading a magazine that you like. You may have to pass up an interesting cover. Boycotting the products of companies who sponsor sexually inappropriate programming has proved a very successful strategy for change. The threat of a boycott often brings results without the necessity of having to organize a national boycott. Local boycotts can be created if the company does not respond; recruit local groups, distribute flyers wherever possible, and involve the media.

The National Coalition on Television Violence (NCTV) screens films and programs and pressures the media to eliminate glorified aggression and violence. It also recommends certain violent films, such as *Born on the Fourth of July,* because the violence portrays the realities of war: The film shows people suffering when violence happens to them. NCTV strongly opposes censorship and publishes a newsletter with its evaluations of the aggressive content of various media depictions. Athough NCTV's job is not to focus only on sexual aggression, the organization does rate films according to their aggressive sexual content, particularly as it relates to children. Some of the films NCTV recommends are highly entertaining and have been very popular.

Books may also influence your ideas, but the average American reads less than one book per year. There is a place for boycotting books. I refuse to buy books written by people who exploit—either those who have committed crimes (Watergate and Irangate government employees have tried to make money this way), or those who expose all of their supposed former lovers in lurid detail. But actually banning books is a dangerous practice, because who is to draw the line? People who attack books are often the same individuals who sit at night with their kids and watch violent shows. The book-banners do not realize where the major harm originates. Opposing books just because you don't like them is like favoring the withdrawal of a medicine whose taste you don't like. You have a perfect right not to buy it. But you need to separate issues of *personal taste* from the *findings of research* before you become alarmed about the media content that you consume. Because books do not show moving images, they are not as compelling to readers as are the visual media.

Call or Write Letters

Protesting a radio or television program is relatively easy. You can call the station and find out the name of the sponsor, producer, or program director. Letters are even more effective. You can note the commercials; if the advertiser's address is not available from the station, a reference librarian can often tell you where to write and protest. Use Ciriello's letter-writing ideas above. Explain what offends you and ask that the offensive show be removed. If it's unsuitable for children, ask that it be moved to a later hour. (See Appendix for a sample letter.)

Note the names of *local* advertisers. Call and politely explain your concerns. Most do not know which shows contain their ads and will be glad to hear your opinions. Be specific and restrict your protests to either aggression or explicit erotic material that is aired at inappropriate times for children. If you merely complain that people's sexual feelings are shocking, you may not be heard.

Thank the Media that Present Entertainment Containing No Sexual Exploitation

Those who support healthy, functional products in the media are jewels. We should value and support them. The publishing house of Simon & Schuster gave up a $300,000 advance to an author whose manuscript was found to be sexually violent. The publishers reportedly discovered that the book would portray a man who tortured and mutilated female victims and adorned his apartment with their body parts. Forty-eight hours after Simon & Schuster decided not to publish, Vintage Books announced their plans to take on the book. The editor of *Publishers Weekly* comments that Vintage has a right to publish it, and the readers have a right to read it. But, he says, " . . . we also care that book publishing should not be so anxious to stay in touch with a perhaps debased popular taste that it abdicates its responsibilities."[10] From such news stories as these, you can find media officials to whom you could make a call or write a letter of appreciation, or a publisher or network whose works you might boycott.

Demonstrate or Picket

Groups often decide to protest by picketing. The way to arrange such a demonstration is to invite other organizations to join you, or call individuals who would be interested in these issues. Print leaflets and posters showing how this show trivializes violence and include quotes from the film, video, or person in question and any statistics from this or other media to support your point. Send press releases to local media at least a week ahead. For a more detailed description of how to demonstrate, see Ciriello's directions in *Transforming a Rape Culture.*[11]

Picketing and demonstrating are nonviolent and legitimate forms of protest. Some people demonstrate for absurd or even evil reasons—such is our constitutional freedom to express our views. But picketing is a courageous and direct way to have an impact. Protesters have picketed shops that rent slasher films, or theaters that pander to sexual violence.

How to Pressure Others to Change the Media

If you want to ask for a new rating system, or warnings, don't bother writing to the motion picture industry. They can use biased surveys to show that parents would rather have the current rating system than nothing, and they have billions to gain from the current competition for the most exploitative films. Instead, you could do the following:

Pressure for New Labeling Systems

Consumers have demanded that food products bear a list of precise contents, and no one considers that pressure to be harassing of the manufacturer. We have a right to know what we're consuming. People get all riled up when they find an unsuspected ingredient in their food or drink: How dare they put something in our food or water without telling us? We should be equally upset if media content is not labeled just as accurately. We should be outraged when unlabeled sexual aggression has been foisted upon us and is desensitizing our entire population.

I have found it personally very frustrating to pay so much for a movie ticket and discover that I have just subsidized sexual aggression. It's discouraging because I am what is often described as a movie freak. But several years ago I began to realize that I was dashing out with enthusiasm to the movies and coming home not just disappointed but troubled. Because of the subjects that I teach, and because of all the survivors who have told me of their pain, I could no longer shut out the exploitation in these films.

I remember when this insight first dawned on me. One summer years ago I attended three films in two weeks. In the first, *Atlantic City,* Burt Lancaster played a character who peered into an apartment window while a woman washed her breasts inside. At first glance this seemed all right because the woman knew he was watching. (Remember that portraying a woman who likes intrusion is the most risky kind of sex in the media.) Later that week I saw *Quest for Fire.* In this film, a primitive woman was raped by a man from another tribe whom she had vehemently disliked. But after the rape she followed him around lovingly and took him for her mate. The third film that week was *Victor/Victoria,* a comedy. Because Julie Andrews's uncertain gender was part of the plot, James Garner hid in a closet to peek at her. Somehow that didn't really seem as if something sexual happened without consent.

There's room for an occasional comedy like *Victor/Victoria.* There's a place for an infrequent drama about rape. But for me it was a shock to realize that *in my country it is hard to find a movie without the little moment of sexual nonconsent.* In the years before and since, we have had major films with nonconsensual sex. It was not always a rape—sometimes just a hint of sexual force was enough to satisfy the moviemakers that they could make money from us. In *Psycho,* a beautiful woman in a shower is stabbed by a crazed madman. In *Stakeout,* the hero who eventually gets the girl hides under her bed and watches her undress. *The Deep* portrays one the bad guys drawing a knife down the very sexy belly of Jacqueline Bisset; will he rape her? We aren't sure. *Pretty Woman,* a big hit, contains a rather prolonged attempted rape. *Ghost,* in the same year, portrays a crazed madman who stumbles upon the lead female and begins to watch her undress, licking his lips, but her cat scares him off. Even *White Palace* has an instance of nonconsensual sex, and almost no one noticed: A young widower, intoxicated, is too drunk to drive home and sleeps at the house of an older woman who is trying to seduce him. He is still grieving over his wife, and he refuses. She implies that she will allow him to sleep it off on her couch, but in the middle of the night she begins to arouse him as he sleeps and her seduction begins a mad, passionate affair. To have sex with someone who is intoxicated and has refused consent qualifies as rape in some states. But since the character likes it, the film once again promotes the belief that *saying no is meaningless.*

In *Rising Sun,* a woman is murdered on a table while moaning in ecstasy during a sexual act. Under the guise of solving the mystery, the film replays her lying there moaning while being murdered, over and over. The mystery part of it is interesting, and I doubt if most people noticed the connection being drilled into their unconscious: Killing is sexy. In *Prince of Tides* there are three rapes, including scary anal rapes of a child. Yet rapes were not always portrayed in such a frightening way. I remember as a child seeing a film called *Johnny Belinda.* I now realize that when the screen went dark in that film it was a signal to adults that there was a rape, but because it was done subtly, it did not frighten me. Those days are gone. Filmmakers amass billions from sexual exploitation. We are being manipulated on a massive scale. Only we can teach filmmakers different attitudes. And only labels can tell us what is in the film before we watch it. Boycotting is our chief way to send a resounding message to the entertainment industry: *We are noticing the nonconsenting sex you are foisting upon us, and we won't buy it.*

Unlike the public acceptance of our inadequate film ratings, an immense controversy has developed about labeling the sexual content of records. For example, 2 Live Crew has recorded a song about a man sexually abusing a woman until she "walks funny." The song says he will break her backbone and "bust her pussy."[12]

NCTV News reports that major songwriters' and publishers' associations have declined or hesitated to oppose the proposed labeling laws, "a clear sign that even people in the recording industry believe things have gone too far."[13]

Our film rating system is not labeling. It is totally inadequate, for rather than listing the "ingredients" the industry decides how appropriate the film is, and they designate it (X, R, NC–17, etc.) for us. They rate it *not according to what is in it* but as a parent would, *according to who can see it.* There exists no real labeling system for television. So many professional groups have concluded that television viewing is one cause of violent or aggressive behavior that there is little disagreement among informed people.

The NCTV has recommended a movie rating system that rates the kind of violence and the harmfulness of the violence. It is based on the idea that ratings should inform people. Their ratings are partially labels—that is, they inform the public about the content of films.

Ask for Prebriefings and Debriefings

Before the movie comes on you hear:

> *What you are about to see depicts people sexually exploiting each other. Research indicates that people who see degrading, insulting, or violent sex may gradually stop feeling shock or disapproval. In addition, other damaging attitude changes can occur in people who view sexually exploitative films. This film also depicts women as willing and eager to participate in any sexual act that a man wants. This view is not accurate. Normal women may like or dislike particular sex acts, and do not always respond enthusiastically to the sexual suggestions of a partner.*

That was a prebriefing—a unique way to decrease the effects of exploitative sex by simply telling the viewer specifically about its harmful effects. Each film or TV piece would include some kind of prebriefing and debriefing at the beginning and end. This information would be more than the kind of warnings that cigarettes and alcohol contain, brief cautions that one can easily ignore. These briefings explain as precisely as possible what the negative effects may be, and they correct myths and other misinformation implied by the film.

Research on sexual aggression shows that people who view it are essentially unaware of its slow but subtle effect on their attitudes. Discussion, however, or listening to a statement about possible harm, can cause attitudes to remain healthier and more rational.[14] A number of studies have found that properly debriefed viewers of a violent rape are not as likely to form the callous view that rape is trivial and common.[15]

We have legally mandated explanations in flyers that accompany drug prescriptions. But because a briefing explains as well as warns, it is quite different from alcohol and cigarette warnings. A *debriefing* could also *follow* a program or film:

> *What you have just seen depicts a woman enjoying a rape. This is not an accurate view. Rape is a serious crime that often causes serious psychological problems in the victim. Rapists can be punished by many years in prison. A common but false belief is that women secretly desire to be raped, or enjoy sexual force. This film also implies that rape is normal for men. Neither of these assumptions is true. Rape is an abnormal act committed more from anger and power than sexual motives. Research shows that watching violent pornography like this may cause viewers to think that sexual violence is less serious than it really is.*

Pre- and *debriefings* will not work if they are a mere canned caution put on all products. They have to be specifically written to neutralize the distorted messages being sent by a particular portrayal. Three of our foremost media researchers recommend that "public service announcements should precede and/or follow television programs that even hint at the justification of violence against women."[16] You say, this will never work? Why not? We now have warnings on cigarettes and alcohol. There is *no proof* that warnings on cigarettes and alcohol actually lessen their harmful effects, but there *is* evidence that prebriefings and debriefings can decrease the damage of exploitative sex in the media. If we knew of a warning that decreased the health risks of cigarettes and alcohol, do you think we should require that it be included on the product? That's how promising prebriefings and debriefings are. And just as medical labels come from medical experts, media labels should be written by experts on aggression in the media. Our goal is to sweep through our entire society with information like the campaigns to inform Americans about the effects of cholesterol or air pollution.

Briefings would not make pornographic material acceptable for children, of course. Regardless of labels or explanations of harm, children should still be protected from watching sexual exploitation of any kind.

Where to Ask for These Changes

If you're determined to influence the portrayal of sex in the media, be prepared to meet people who might seem appallingly different from you. Although you may see aggression as the major issue, others may view explicit sex as the culprit. It is unquestionably a bit of a strain to join ranks with someone who is miles away from you philosophically. But many successful political alliances in this country have been made by people willing to ignore differences that are irrelevant to their goals.

Write Your Legislators

Make sure your state senators and representatives and your U.S. senators and representatives in Congress are aware of a few research facts along with your views. (If you need to know their names and addresses, call the League of Women Voters in your area.) Ask for accurate labeling and explain prebriefings and debriefings. Explain any intentions you may have to vote against politicians who fail to support the issues you value.

Search for Organizations to Support

Join or contribute to national organizations that agree with your views. Put your money where your mouth is. Choose carefully from your own contacts or from the organizations listed in the Appendix. Join local groups that are active in demanding labeling and rating changes. Recruit people to help from churches and temples, PTAs, and other community groups. The Junior League has been very effective in this battle. If there is a Junior League in your area, call and find out what you can do. Be prepared to pursue the subject through a number of phone calls.

Support Conflict Resolution Training Everywhere

Schools, churches, temples, and workplaces can teach the skills that we should have learned in a peaceful tribe and family. There are consultants who can prepare children and adults to use these skills.

Complain to the FCC

Write or call the Federal Communications Commission to complain, make suggestions, or urge that the FCC require high-quality children's program of an educational and instructional nature as a condition of license renewal for television stations. (See Appendix for the address of the FCC.)

Speaking Up for Children

There is no question that childhood influences can stay with us for life. Children can learn permanent attitudes as early as birth; I have even known several people born with the umbilical cord around their necks who as adults could not bear to wear turtlenecks or mufflers but had never made the connection. The immature brain has an awesome ability to latch onto experiences and learn permanent attitudes or emotions from these events. Our society allows very harmful influences during children's most sensitive developmental years. Most of our struggles with ourselves involve getting past the past. Childhood is the foundation on which the adult personality is formed, and invariably therapists find that sex offenders suffer from early influences.

But children don't just absorb unhealthy attitudes from the family. The more sick a society, the more distorted attitudes form in the average child. If we care about our society, we will do all we can to protect its children. In a real sense, *they are ours.*

How to Report Child Abuse

Abusing a child physically or sexually is one of the principal ways to set a human being on the path of victimizing others. Although some survivors escape without ever becoming abusers, most sex offenders have been abused either sexually or physically. It's hard to believe that an innocent little child could grow up to hurt other people. But it happens frequently.

Suspecting child abuse automatically creates a responsibility. *You may be the only person in the world who suspects that this child is being abused and who can defend him.* Don't buy into the fear of being a tattletale—that is just a hangover from elementary school. Don't let the child down; if you even suspect any form of abuse, call your state's child abuse hotline. If you're concerned about anonymity or procedures, check with the hotline beforehand.

Supervising Television

The most dysfunctional families—whose children are the *most* susceptible to media influence—are the *least* likely families to supervise TV. It is absurd to think that most parents screen what their children watch. Some don't even care if their kids are on drugs, much less whether they are being sexualized. Many others care but are too preoccupied with problems. And what kind of sense does it make to put a powerfully attractive box in the living room and then tell children not to watch? If drug companies sold delicious, eye-catching medicines in bottles with no safety lids, we would be up in arms. We should be equally concerned about attractive but potentially harmful media presentations that our children can watch with no constraints.

Whenever you view any form of exploitative or aggressive sex in the presence of a child, you have a chance to do your own editorializing. The child should preferably not watch harmful programs. But if something damaging comes on television unexpectedly, you can interrupt the kids' program:

"I don't like to hear people laugh and call each other bad names. Sometimes we get mad at each other, but we don't call each other bad names." (Or, if you're speaking to a teenager,) "I really get upset over this program. What do you think would happen if people really treated each other like this? They make it look like people can't solve any problems without hurting someone. What do you think?"

You can editorialize (debrief) about pornography as well. Norma Ramos, the general counsel for Women Against Pornography, says that parents must become aware of how to influence children not to participate in this epidemic of sexual exploitation. "We have to stop socializing boys the way we do," she says. "When parents see their sons reading pornography, they should engage them in a *real* serious dialogue. What are the messages that are being sent to your son?"[17]

I suggest that if you find your little brother or your child reading any sexually degrading material, even if it is nonviolent and merely makes women look like idiot playthings, you comment: "I notice you're reading . . . . What do you think about that?" He'll probably say: "Nothin'." You could say: "You know why I don't like to see you looking at this stuff? Because people aren't really like this, this isn't what normal people do. This magazine makes women look like playthings, and men look like they are just using women. Healthy relationships are a lot different. . . . "

You can elaborate according to your views and how extreme the material is. Remember, you're not just whistling in the wind. There is solid research to indicate that when you make remarks about a program, you can change attitudes in adults or children. You are *debriefing*. I hope you don't let any opportunities pass. Research evidence also indicates that when there is no adult commenting to the contrary, children tend to think what they're doing is okay.

Press for a Children's TV Network

Miriam Miedzian proposes an exciting and encouraging direction for giving children healthy entertainment:[18]

> *We need two public television channels dedicated to top quality, nonviolent, pro-social programming—one for young children, roughly aged two to nine; another for preadolescents aged ten to thirteen. . . . The creation of a children's public television network would be a sign of deep societal concern for the wellbeing of children and the curbing of violence. . . . The creation of a viable CPBS will require a long-range congressional commitment to ongoing funding. . . .*

Support Involved Fathers

Boys find out how to be men from adult males. They need to see men who have empathy, because such men do not exploit people. Callous, macho males are greatly lacking in this basic human ability to understand how someone else feels. A 26-year longitudinal study of boys found that the single factor most closely linked to empathy and concern for others was the level of their fathers' involvement in their care.[19] Where large groups of fatherless boys congregate, gangs and violence often arise to fulfill the enormous void in which a father's presence would tell these boys how to be men. Support fathers' involvement in child care and family life in all possible ways.

Insist on Education

We know that classes about the influences of media can educate even our youngest schoolchildren. Prebriefing educational messages can alert viewers to the seriousness of the violence they are about to witness. Thorough sex education programs in all schools can prepare young people to cope with their sexuality and to understand how their culture is distorting their sexual attitudes. Excellent rape- and harassment-prevention programs are in place in a few high schools and colleges. If we don't want censorship, we are going to have to have an educated population.

One reason parents are scared about sex education is that they don't know what values the teachers are going to impart to their children. There are some issues, such as abortion, that are so controversial no program addressing the subject would ever pass the current political climate. Why not leave out abortion and agree on the basics of health education? In addition to the biological facts, all children should learn the skills of resisting sexual pressure—how to avoid molestation in the early years and use sexual assertiveness in all the years following. All children, even before they are old enough to get into sexual trouble, should learn about disease and pregnancy prevention as well as the reasons they are too young for sex. And yet, the skillful teacher can still avoid making sex sound like a scary thing; the approach should stress planning and responsibility.

If some teachers don't know how to do that, we must find the funds for more teacher training. Excellent teachers can put sexual safety in a wise and cautious context. Parents often fear that, by discussing sex openly and honestly, teachers will encourage sexual activity. The research does not bear out this fear. A skilled teacher can avoid *endorsing* premarital sex, but can teach about disease and pregnancy as subjects students will need to know at some point in their lives. We do, after all, teach about many things that students may not immediately use.

Encouraging studies show that we can prevent the media from damaging our children through *specific* educational techniques. If our society is going to be warped enough to besiege its children with exploitative messages, the least we can do is arm them with healthy attitudes to help them withstand the assault.

To exert pressure for better health education, try to work out programs where people with various beliefs may choose options for their children, perhaps through levels of sex education. In middle school and high school this plan could begin with an already established and successful program, Postponing Sexual Involvement.[20] Emphasize the concern we all have in common: the sexual safety and responsibility of our young people.

Be of Good Courage

Don't expect immediate change in everything you attempt. Feel good right now that you're taking a stand. Be proud of yourself for that. It may take time for various inroads to be made, but they are beginning already.

If You Add Your Voice

Sandra Campbell writes compellingly about using the power of our voices to heal the harm from centuries of violence. She writes, " . . . Each of us, informed by our heads and our hearts, can use our voices as primary instruments and can become the agents for transforming our culture by creating images that foster hope for ourselves and our future."[21] It is vital that you find your voice. When you assert yourself or disagree in person with other people's opinions, you may feel embarrassed at first because of the people who are present. But you should feel proud. Remember the survivors and potential victims who are not there. For just as a friend thanks you for defending her in her absence, if you could hear the voices of millions of survivors, you would hear them say thank you. Thank you for speaking up so that what I have suffered may be even partially vindicated. Thank you for ensuring that all of us have less chance of being hurt in the future. Thank you.

Although I am a college professor and have tried to present objective data here, this book is not an academic treatise: It is a formula for action. I could not have written these words with such conviction had I not been fueled with the determination of a woman, a mother, a friend and loved one of survivors, and an American who cares that my society should endure and prosper.

It is not a favor to society when we speak up. It is our obligation. Those who will inherit our earth and our society deserve to be protected. I share the belief of Native Americans that the earth is a sacred trust, and we must leave it as safe as we found it. A healthy society is also a sacred trust—we should not allow it to be damaged. We owe to future generations a safe place in which to grow.

In the words of the Talmud,

I did not find this world desolate when I entered it.
My ancestors planted for me before I was born.
So do I plant for those who come after me.

Debrief Your Friends After the Movie

Look for one of the sexual messages you have just checked in the TV assignment on pages 194–195. Or, assume the following:

You and your friends have just seen a movie that depicts some cute guys peeping in on a woman getting dressed. At another point in the movie a man pushes a woman into sex while she's saying no, and suddenly in the middle of this she begins loving it. On the outside it looks like just another entertaining movie, but your consciousness is raised and you realize there are two incidents of sex without consent. You know from research that films showing women fighting off men and suddenly loving it can subtly change the attitudes of your friends, especially if no one disagrees. Debrief your friends by informing them of your objections to this movie. Try to put the comments into your own words:

That movie we just saw. . . I felt . . . when that movie showed . . .

Respond to These Jokes

You are in a crowd that keeps making jokes putting down people of your gender. They either make fun of how "You know how all men are," or they tell jokes that generalize about women. You're beginning to feel uncomfortable just sitting there letting them think you don't mind. You say, "I feel very . . . when I hear jokes about. . . . ." Or say something more original, using your own words.

You are in a mixed group sitting in a restaurant. Someone tells a joke:

Question: What do 30,000 abused women have in common?

Answer: They just wouldn't listen.

   1. How do you think you would really respond?

   a. Laugh
   b. Tell them the joke is sexist
   c. Make a slightly displeased face and change the subject
   d. Preserve a stony silence

   2. How do you think you *should* respond? Choose one of the following or write your own response:

   a. "I don't like jokes that make fun of hurting people."
   b. "You guys are jerks."
   c. "I'm out of here."
   d. _____

Notes

1. From a union protest song of the same title. Copyright 1947, People's Songs, in *Songs of Work and Freedom* (Garden City, N.Y. Doubleday and Company, 1960), 54.

2. Donna Eder and Janet Lynne Erke, "The Structure of Gossip: Opportunities and

Constraints on Collective Expression in Adolescents. *American Sociological Review* 56 (1991): 494–508.

3. As cited by Elizabeth Powell, "I Thought You Didn't Mind," in Buchwald, Fletcher, and Roth, eds., *Transforming a Rape Culture,* 116.

4. Norman Cousins, *Head First: The Biology of Hope and the Healing Power of the Human Spirit* (New York: Penguin Books, 1989).

5. D. Linz, J. Niemczycki, and E. Donnerstein, "The Effects of Co-viewing Spectators on Perceptions of Sexual Violence." Unpublished manuscript, University of California at Santa Barbara, 1990.

6. Linz, Niemczycki, and Donnerstein, "The Effects of Co-viewing Spectators on Perceptions of Sexual Violence," 160.

7. Powell, "I Thought You Didn't Mind," in Buchwald, Fletcher, and Roth, eds., *Transforming a Rape Culture,* 116.

8. Sarah Ciriello, "Commodification of Women: Morning, Noon, and Night," in Buchwald, Fletcher, and Roth, eds., *Transforming a Rape Culture,* 276.

9. Ciriello, "Commodification of Women," in Buchwald, Fletcher, and Roth, eds., *Transforming a Rape Culture,* 277.

10. John N. Baker, "Publisher Responsibility and Bret Easton Ellis," *Publishers Weekly,* 30 November 1990, 7.

11. Ciriello, "Commodification of Women," Buchwald, Fletcher, and Roth, eds., *Transforming a Rape Culture,* 277–278.

12. "As Nasty as They Wanna Be," Luke Records, PAC JAM Publishing (BMI), Liberty City, Fla.

13. Radecki, *NCTV News,* 2.

14. Daniel Linz et al., "Bases of Liability for Injuries Produced by Media Portrayals of Violent Pornography," in Malamuth and Donnerstein, eds., *Pornography and Sexual Aggression,* 277–304.

15. J. V. P. Check and N. M. Malamuth, "Can Exposure to Pornography Have Positive Effects?" Paper presented at the annual meeting of the American Psychological Association, Los Angeles, August 1981.

16. Donnerstein, Linz, and Malamuth, *The Question of Pornography,* 195–196.

17. Telephone interview, July 19, 1990.

18. Miedzian, *Boys Will Be Boys,* 234–240.

19. Richard Koestner, Carol Franz, and Joel Weinberger, "The Family Origins of Empathic Concern: A 26-year Longitudinal Study," *Journal of Personality and Social Psychology* (1990): 709–717, as cited by Miedzian, *Boys Will Be Boys.*

20. Information on this program can be obtained from Grady Memorial Hospital, Emory/Grady Teen Services Program, Hospital Box 26158, 80 Butler Street S.E., Atlanta, GA 30335.

21. Sandra Campbell, "Creating Redemptive Imagery," Buchwald, Fletcher, and Roth, eds., *Transforming a Rape Culture,* 151.

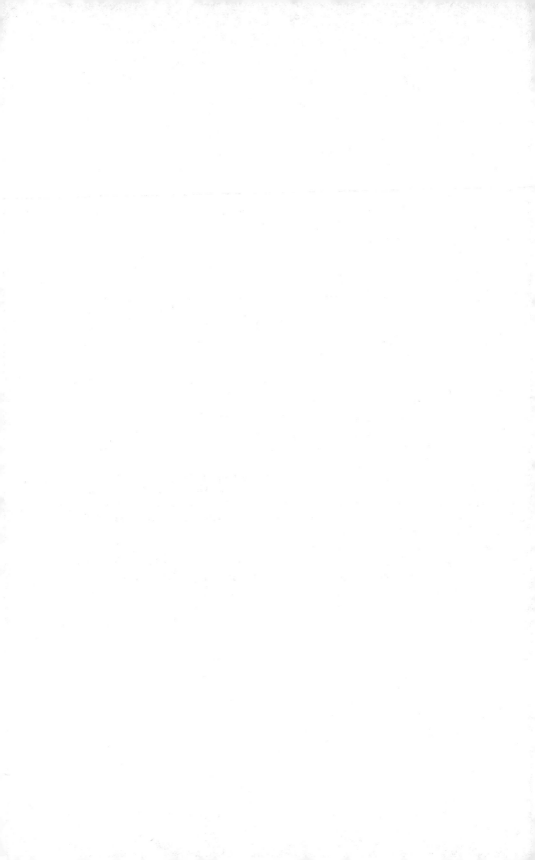

Appendix

Remember that you should apply basic good judgment in choosing an organization, agency, or therapist, or in deciding on actions to ensure your safety. You will need to take responsibility for checking out any sources listed here. You may be able to call one of these sources to get information about others not listed. You'd be surprised at what I've found out doing that. Keep asking. You might say, for example: "I'm trying to find some help with . . . and I haven't been able to find anything. Do you know of an agency or person who could help me? Or someone who might know about that subject? Is there anyone in your agency who might have some ideas?"

Large libraries usually have phone directories from every major city. Even if you're trying to assist someone long distance, looking through the yellow pages can aid you in finding help for psychological, medical, religious, and other problems.

If you live in a small town and cannot find local resources, try the largest nearby city. Have your list of questions by the phone when you call to ask about services, confidentiality, fees, etc. Don't be embarrassed to call back if you think of another question.

Because of the low priority of these issues in our society, privately supported agencies sometimes lose funding. If you call a number that is no longer in service, try dialing information. In other cases, phone lines that take complaints can jam, so keep trying.

Preventing Sexual Aggression in the Media

Organizations to Join

Here are two well-known groups working hard against exploitation. Neither group advocates censorship:

National Coalition on Television Violence, c/o Dr. Robert E. Gould, 144 East End Ave., New York, NY 10028, 1-212-535-7275; Women Against Pornography, P.O. Box 845, Times Square Station, New York, NY 10036, 1-212-307-5055. There are also several other organizations that act as watchdog groups to urge changes in the media; most are religiously affiliated. To find one, ask your librarian.

Where to Send Protest Letters, Suggestions, or Complaints

> *Complaints and Investigation Bureau,*
> *TV, Radio, and Cable Complaints*
> *Federal Communications Commission*
> *2025 M Street NW, Room 8202*
> *Washington, DC 20554; 1-202-418-1430*
>
> *Fox TV Center*
> *5746 W. Sunset Blvd.*
> *Los Angeles, CA 90028*
>
> *NBC*
> *30 Rockefeller Plaza*
> *New York, NY 10112*
>
> *CBS*
> *51 W. 52nd Street*
> *New York, NY 10019*
>
> *ABC*
> *47 W. 66th Street*
> *New York, NY 10023*

Sample Protest Letter

A letter should be brief and might go something like this:

> *Dear (sponsor, network or local station, business, etc.),*
>
> *Yesterday I watched a program (or saw a commercial or an advertisement) (on your station, on your network, or sponsored by your company) that I found very offensive. It occurred on (date, time, station, channel) and it depicted (mention any kind of aggression to which you object.) I enclose a copy of the objectionable ad (if possible).*
> *Research shows that portraying . . . can be harmful, even to adults. Once in every fifteen seconds a woman is beaten up by a man in this coun-*

try, but your ad shows a man doing . . . . I do not want my (brothers, sons) watching this kind of degrading material.

I am hoping you will reconsider this (ad, program, etc.) in light of our serious national problems with these kinds of aggression and violence. It would be more socially responsible for you to (advertise, etc.) in other ways.

(Option): If necessary, I plan to organize a boycott against your (products, network, business) until such time as you cease to sponsor sexually exploitative or violent material. I am sending copies of this letter to (mention target groups, media, etc.) (Or): This is not the kind of programming that I want (my family) to watch. I hope that you upgrade your programming so that viewers can see exciting content that is not violent.

Sincerely,

Disease Prevention and Birth Control

Sources of Information and/or Testing

These services should always be confidential, but you may want to double-check to feel reassured. There are some state laws requiring the reporting of certain STDs to keep track for health purposes.

Planned Parenthood has centers in most major cities in the U.S. and offers contraception and other services, depending on the center. Check your phone book for the number. *County health departments* usually provide sites for testing and treatment for STDs. Look in your phone book or ask the operator. You may want to inquire about the people to whom the testing site reports results, and the confidentiality of those results, especially in testing for the HIV (AIDS) virus. There are some slight differences in the way this is handled, and HIV-positive individuals are rightly concerned about confidentiality.

AIDS prevention and AIDS support groups have sprung up in various locations and can refer you to testing sources. Check your phone book for AIDS agencies to get a referral.

Hotlines

National STD Hotline: 1-800-227-8922
National AIDS Hotline: 1-800-342-AIDS
    For Hispanics: 1-800-344-SIDA
    For the deaf: 1-800-243-7889
    National Herpes Hotline: 1-919-361-8488

To order a book about herpes, call 1-800-783-9877

For a unique pamphlet about hygiene practices that can decrease the risk of STD, send $1: American Foundation for the Prevention of Venereal Disease, Inc., 799 Broadway, Suite 638, New York, NY 10003.

For information on how to use a condom correctly, or to learn about high-and low-risk behaviors for any STD: Call government-sponsored testing sites listed under your county's health department, or Planned Parenthood, or the STD or the AIDS hotline (above), or your college health service.

In case of sexual harassment, the two major agencies are: Equal Employment Opportunity Commission (check the government section of your phone book) and the Human Rights Commission (check your state capitol for the number). The Feminist Majority runs a sexual harassment hotline in Washington, DC: 1-703-522-2501.

TABLE App.1   Legal Assistance for Sexual Harrassment and Sexual Assault

Name	Description	How to Locate
Title VII—Civil Rights Act	Federal legislation prohibiting sex discrimination in employment	EEOC: Equal Employment Opportunity Commission
State Civil Rights Laws	Similar to Title VII, but vary from state to state	Your state's human rights commission
Title IX—Education Amendments	Prohibits sex discrimination in education	OCR: Office of Civil Rights, Dept. of Education (regional offices)
Criminal Rape Statutes	Vary among states; some laws include degrees of sexual assault other than forcible rape. Apply *only* when actual assault occurs	Police or prosecuting attorney
Other Criminal Charges	Assault, battery, or intentional infliction of emotional harm	Police or prosecuting attorney
Civil Lawsuit	Private money damages, but very difficult to get unless actual physical assault	Private attorney
Workers Compensation	Some states beginning to recognize claims for emotional distress arising from sexual harrassment by employer	Private attorney

Help For Children

To Report Child Abuse

Most states have a child abuse hotline. To find yours, call information or the operator. Or call the National Child Abuse Hotline, 1–800–4-A-CHILD. Runaways are often running from sexual abuse at home. The National Runaway Switchboard is: 1-800-621-4000.

Help for Violence at Home

Center for the Prevention of Sexual and Domestic Violence, 1914 N. 34th St., Suite 105, Seattle, WA 98103, 1-206-634-1903.

Help for Alcohol and Drug Abuse

For the Addict

Check your phone book or in the next largest town for the National Council on Alcohol and Drug Abuse, Alcoholics Anonymous, and Narcotics Anonymous.

For Family or a Friend

Those who care about someone affected by alcohol and/or drug abuse can call Al-Anon or Al-Ateen. If you do not find the number in the phone book, call your local Alcoholics Anonymous chapter.

Drug Hotlines:

The number for Al-Anon Family Group Headquarters is 1-800-356-9996. There is also a Cocaine Hotline that answers questions and provides treatment referrals: 1-800-COCAINE. The National Institute on Drug Abuse has a Drug Abuse Information and Referral Line: 1-800-662-4357.

Help for Survivors of Sexual Exploitation

In big cities you should look in the phone book for the people who could most logically refer you for help: the rape crisis hotline or any kind of women's center (which is often on a college or university campus). They may know where to refer male survivors as well. If you're in a small town, call long distance; many women's centers will let you reverse the charges.

Incest

Two organizations that help provide support groups nationwide for incest survivors are Survivors of Incest Anonymous, P.O. Box 21817, Baltimore, MD 21222-6817, 1-410-282-3400; and Incest Survivors Anonymous, P.O. Box 5613, Long Beach, CA 90805-0613, 1-310-428-5599.

There are a number of books available for survivors. Ask one of the above groups for suggestions.

Preventing and Treating Rape

Rape crisis hotlines exist in almost all major cities. They are sometimes listed as a crisis hotline. Ask the operator for the number, or call a county- or state-run counseling department. If you are in a small town, get the information operator in a large city and call a crisis hotline long distance; they may let you call collect. You might get further information from the National Clearinghouse on Marital and Date Rape, 2325 Oak Street, Berkeley, CA 94708, 1-510-524-1582, or Women Organized Against Rape, 1233 Locust Street, Suite 2102, Philadelphia, PA 19107, 1-215-922-7400.

Your Personal Safety Checklist to Prevent Stranger Rape:

Check those things you do routinely:

At Home

___ I refuse to admit anyone to my home or apartment that I do not know or was not expecting.

___ I always ask to see proper identification through a closed door or peephole.

___ I leave the door open if a properly identified repairman enters, and plan where I would go if the situation became threatening.

___ I list my name by initials only on my mailbox and in the phone book.

___ I always keep my doors and windows locked.

___ I use timers to turn on lights and radio if I expect to be out all day.

___ I have the key ready before I approach my car or my home.

___ I have adequate lighting at all doors.

___ I have a phone by my bed.

___ I vary my routine a little each day if I have to be in a risky area.

___ I do not allow strangers to use my phone.

In the Car

___ I keep my car, tires, etc., in good condition to prevent breakdown.

___ I keep my car doors and windows locked at all times.

___ I travel on well-lighted streets where people are always around.

___ I have plans to stay in my car if it breaks down.

___ I carry a SEND HELP sign.

___ I have a quarter taped to a card with a tow truck number so that I can pass it through a window crack.

___ I keep the car in gear while waiting at a stop sign.

___ I check the rear view mirror occasionally and know where to find police, fire station, or other safe place if I am followed.

___ I remember to sound the horn if I need to get attention.

___ I try to park my car where it is well lighted at night.

___ I lock my car at all times and look inside before unlocking it.

___ Whenever possible, at night I walk out of shopping centers, work, or other places along with other people.

In Public Places

___ I use drugs little if at all; my drug use allows me to remain in control.

___ I drive my own car or arrange a ride so that I needn't depend on someone I do not know well.

___ If I am harassed by a person in a public place, such as a bar, I report him to the owner, bouncer, or bartender.

___ I walk near the street and avoid places such as alleys, doorways, or shrubbery where someone could hide.

___ If a driver pulls over to ask directions, I call them out briefly from a safe distance.

___ I do not hitchhike under any circumstances.

___ I do not walk alone at night.

___ I wear shoes that allow me to run if necessary.

___ I am prepared to approach a house for help.

___ I carry a loud siren, a whistle, or a buzzer for attracting attention in an emergency.

___ I am prepared, if a car approaches me and the driver threatens me, to scream and run in the opposite direction from the car.

___ I walk with my head up and with confidence as if I know where I am going.

___ If I find myself on an elevator with someone who seems risky, I get off at the next floor; if such a person enters an elevator I am planning to enter, I wait until the empty elevator returns.

___ I always stand near the control panel on an elevator so that I can reach the alarm if necessary.

Immediately After a Rape:

1. Don't change anything about your body—don't wash or even comb your hair. Leave your clothes as they are. You could destroy evidence.

2. Strongly consider reporting the incident to police. You may prevent another woman from being assaulted, and you will be taking charge, starting the path from victim to survivor.

3. Ask a relative or friend to take you to a hospital; if you can't, get an ambulance or a police car. If you call the hospital, tell them why you're requesting an ambulance; they might send someone trained in rape crisis.

4. Seeking help is an assertive way to show you're worth it. Seek medical help even if you don't intend to report the rape to the police. Injuries of which you are unaware may be detected. Insist that a written or photographic record be made documenting your condition. You may decide later that you're going to prosecute, and you'll need evidence.

5. You have medical rights. Ask questions. Ask what's available to you, ask for what you need to make you comfortable. You are calling the shots now. Ask for confidentiality if that's what you want. Refuse what you don't want.

A Book for Rape Survivors:
Quest for Respect, by Linda Braswell (Pathfinder Publishing of California, 458 Dorothy Ave., Ventura, CA 93003, 1990). A very short book that takes you step by step through recovery. There are a number of other books available. Ask your local library or bookstore.

Sources of Help for Sex Offenders

Organizations:

These are often listed in the white pages of large urban phone directories. Or write the national offices for information about the closest group: Sex Addicts Anonymous, P.O. Box 70949, Houston, Texas 77270; Sexaholics Anonymous (Sex Addiction), P.O. Box 300, Simi Valley, CA 93062.

A helpful book is *Contrary to Love: Helping the Sexual Addict,* by Patrick Carnes, Ph.D. (Minneapolis: CompCare, 1989).

If You Need Psychotherapy

Good counseling or psychotherapy can improve your self-esteem, help you recover from past traumatic experiences, and reach your best potential. This effort requires a search on your part. If you've been victimized by a man, you may want to start with a woman therapist and vice versa. Try asking for a referral from one of the following:

- a crisis hotline
- a women's center on a college or university campus
- a local mental health association
- a counselor at your high school or college
- one of the other contacts listed in this Appendix

Don't continue with the first counselor you meet if you have major doubts about the person. The counselor should be supportive, yet try to help you to become self-sufficient so that you can deal with your problems constructively. Look for a professional therapist licensed with other credentials at the Master's degree level or beyond, and experience. An emotionally stable therapist welcomes questions about training or qualifications. She may be accredited by organizations at which you could double-check her credentials. The therapist should be objective—not a friend, not a lover. She should do more than just listen; she should help *you* to define your issues and be the active problem solver in your own life. Don't be afraid to get a second opinion from another therapist if you are not sure you've chosen someone suitable for you. Some people work better with certain kinds of clients.

To get further referrals, send a self-addressed, stamped envelope to the National Self-Help Clearinghouse, 25 West 43rd Street, New York, New York 10036. If you want to find a national support group, you could call NSHC at 1-212-354-8525.

United Way (or United Fund) in many major cities often has a referral number that connects people with sources of help for all kinds of problems. Look in the white business pages of your phone book.

Research Data on Alcohol and Sexual Risk

In Chapter 5 there is a questionnaire about sexual risks and alcohol in your life. Various other surveys of college and university students were combined by Kathy Kodama at the University of California at Berkeley (printed in the National

Collegiate AIDS Network Newsletter, No. 5, January 30, 1991, p. 4). The results below also show a combined score from my three human sexuality classes in the fall of 1994 at St. Louis Community College:

The following percentages of each sample answered *True* to the questions on pp. 104–105, Chapter 5:

1. Kodama, 15 percent of the women, 17 percent of men (This was the only instance in which men and women were considered separately.)
   Powell, 21 percent
2. Kodama, 62 percent
   Powell, 48 percent
3. Kodama, 42 percent
   Powell, 33 percent
4. Kodama, 14 percent
   Powell, 40 percent
5. Kodama, 44 percent
   Powell, 48 percent
6. Kodama, 38 percent
   Powell, 37 percent
7. Kodama, 47 percent
   Powell, 35 percent

(Items 8 and 9 from p. 105 were not on the above surveys.)

Index

Abortion, 98–99
Abstinence, 60–65
Acquaintance rape, 138–157
  alcohol use and, 24, 142, 143, 146, 151
  by ex-boyfriends, 147, 168
  help immediately after, 153–154, 228
  legal issues concerning, 134, 145, 151,
    154, 161
  male justification of, 149–150
  male responsibility for preventing, 8,
    150–152
  mixed messages and, 18, 140, 141, 147,
    149–150
  and obscene phone calls, 169
  prevention of, 8, 145–148, 150–152
  rapist characteristics, 141–145
  statutory, by helping professionals, 18,
    129
  See also Rape
Acquired Immune Deficiency Syndrome
    (AIDS), 3
  abstinence and, 62
  and beliefs about health, 39
  risk of acquiring, 5, 79–83, 86, 88, 99
Affirmations, 36, 45–46
Aggression. See Sexual aggression
Alcohol use, 24–25
  family scripts and, 33
  help for, 20, 225
  rape and, 24, 142, 143, 146, 151
  as risk trigger, 84, 229–230

American Academy of Pediatrics, 180
American Medical Association, 180
American Psychological Association, 180
Anal sex, 99
Anger, 8, 9, 15–16, 33, 147–148
Antisocial personality disorders, 20
Arousal, 15–16, 65–66
Assertiveness training, 11–12
Attitudes
  beliefs and, 34–37, 60–65
  changing, techniques for, 41–42, 45–47
  courage, 40, 92, 144, 217
  depression and, 44–45
  family scripts and, 33–34, 42–44, 47
  importance of, 29–30
  and mind versus body, 32–33
  policy statement in, 58–61, 73–74, 90,
    91, 145–146
  rewards and, 38–40
  self-esteem and, 38–40, 68, 95–96,
    114–115
  See also Cultural messages
Attorney General's Commission on
    Pornography, 180
Attorneys, sexual harassment by, 130

Behavioral Group Intervention to Teach
    AIDS Reduction Skills (Kelly and St.
    Lawrence), 57–58
Beliefs, 34–37, 60–65
Birth control devices, 97

Birth control pills, 53, 62, 83, 97, 98
Boasting, 24, 67–68
Body language, 20–21, 117
Books
brainwashing and, 53–54
sexual violence in, 4, 18, 136–137
Boycotts, product, 207–208
Boys Will Be Boys (Miedzian), 191–192
Brainwashing, 53–54, 66–69, 178
Braswell, Linda, 153
Burke, Edmund, 200
Butler, Pamela, 36

Calderone, Mary, 161
Campbell, Sandra, 217
Carlson, Nancy, 140
Casual sex, 99–100
Censorship, 179
Centers for Disease Control, 79, 83, 101
Cervical cancer, 63
Challenging Media Images of Women Newsletter, 205
Cheating, 66
Chemical dependency, 24–25
Child abuse, 17, 214, 225
Children, 213–216
family scripts and, 33–34, 42–44, 47
and involvement of fathers, 215–216
parental influence on, 33–34, 42–44, 47
and pretend-love relationships, 62–63
puberty, changes in, 19
safety of, 3, 9, 19
sex education and, 19, 216
sexual abuse of, 3, 152, 161
sexual assertiveness for, 9
sexual rights of, 19
television and, 214–215
Chlamydia, 80–82, 102
Ciriello, Sarah, 205, 208, 209
Civil Rights Act of 1964, Title VII, 127
Clarke, Elissa, 123
Clothing rights, 18–19, 118, 141, 149, 163–164
Cocaine, 24–25
Coercion, sexual, 160–162. *See also* Acquaintance rape; Rape

Complaints
about media messages, 205–211, 222–223
about sexual harassment, 124–126
about sexual intrusion, 172–173
Compulsive sexuality. *See* Sexual addiction
Condoms
attitudes toward use of, 31
discussion of, 17, 42, 87–98
safety of, 86, 94–95, 97–98
stopping use of, 83, 85, 99
Conflict resolution skills, 213
Confrontive assertion, 13–14
Contraception
discussion of, 17, 35
failure to use, 7–8, 31
information on, 223
sharing expenses of, 17
See also Birth control pills; Condoms
Counseling, 130, 152, 153
Courage, 40, 92, 144, 217
Cousins, Norman, 201
Cultural messages, 30–32
abstinence and, 61–62
and customs of sexual pressure, 51–53
men and, 30–31
rape and, 134–141, 164, 179
sexual confusion, 58–59
women and, 31–32
See also Mass media

Date rape. *See* Acquaintance rape
Davis, Margaret, 102–103
Debriefings, movie, 212, 215
Demonstrations, protest, 208–209
Denial, 85
Dentists, sexual harassment by, 129–130
Depression, 44–45, 114, 129, 152
Desensitization, 182
Disappointment, 16
Double binds, 68–69
Drug use, 24–25, 225

Eders, Donna, 200
Ellis, Albert, 35
Empathic assertion, 12–13

Employment
  clothing rights and, 18–19, 118
  sexual harassment and, 5, 8, 18,
    109–112, 123
  sexual rights and, 18
Erotica, 183–185
Escalating assertion, 13
Ethics
  of helping professionals, 18, 128–130
  sexual, 15–19, 56–57, 66, 93, 152
Exhibitionism, 8, 17, 160, 170, 172, 201
Explicit sex, 184
Eye contact, 117, 162–165

Familiarity, 143–145
Family scripts, 33–34, 42–44, 47
Fantasies
  dangerous, 17
  guided imagery and, 41
  sexual, 16–17, 160
Fathers, involvement of, 215–216
Federal Communications Commission
  (FCC), 213
First Amendment, 179
Flashers, 170
Foreplay, 103
Fraternity Gang Rape (Sanday), 138
Frustration, 16, 61, 66

Game playing, 15–16, 33, 68–69
Gang rape, 138, 178
Gay bashing, 3
Genital herpes, 80–82, 86, 102
Genital warts, 80–82
Gonorrhea, 80–82, 102
Gordon, Sol, 56
Gossip, 200
Government
  censorship by, 179
  research on impact of violence in media,
    180
Guided imagery, 41
Guilt, arousal and, 15–16, 65–66

Harassment, *see* Sexual harassment.
Helping professionals
  ethical standards of, 18, 128–130

sexual harassment by, 128–130
  statutory rape and, 18, 129
Herpes, genital, 80–82, 86, 102
HIV, 45, 79, 82, 99, 100, 101, 102
Holistic approach, 46–47
Honesty, 19–20, 56–57, 93, 152
Hotlines, 83, 99, 101, 129, 153, 154 (also
  see Appendix)
Howard, Marion, 63–64
Human immunodeficiency virus (HIV)
  risky practices and, 83, 85, 99
  testing for, 101
  See also Acquired Immune Deficiency
    Syndrome (AIDS)
Human Sexuality (Masters and Johnson),
  6–7
Humor
  connection with aggression in media,
    137, 180–181
  exploitive jokes and, 4, 18, 123, 201–203
  rape and, 137
  in responding to sexual pressure,
    56
Hypnosis, self-, 45–46

Incest
  double binds in, 68–69
  support groups for, 46–47, 226
  survivors of, 177–178, 226
I Never Called it Rape (Warshaw),
  141–143, 144
In Love and Friendship (Norman), 136
Intimacy, abstinence and, 62, 64
Intrusion, *see* Sexual intrusion.
I-statements, 21–24, 121, 122

Jakubowski, Patricia, 12–14
Jealousy, 142, 144
Johnson, Virginia E., 6–7
Jokes, 4, 18, 123, 201–203

Kama Sutra, 183
Kelly, Jeffrey, 57–58, 99–100
Kimmel, Michael S., 140
Kissing, 100, 184
Klein, Marty, 4
Koss, Mary, 137–138

Lange, Arthur J., 12–14
Language, sexual, 7
Lecherous Professor, The (Dziech and
  Weiner), 120
Leering, 110, 162–165
Legal issues
  rape and, 134, 145, 151, 154, 161
  sexual harassment and, 18, 127, 224
  sexually transmitted diseases and,
    102–103
Legal issues, *continued*
  stalking and, 171–172
Letters, 125–126, 208
"Locker-room bragging," 24, 67–68
Loneliness, abstinence and, 64
Love, 19, 44–45, 56, 62–63, 63
Lovers, Doctors, and the Law (Davis),
  102–103
Lying, 22, 93

Macho personality, 191–192, 205
Madhubuti, Haki, 152
Magazines, sexual violence in, 4
Malamuth, Neil, 141
Marijuana, 24–25
Marital rape, 134, 178
Marshall, W. L., 188
Masculinity
  attitudes toward, 4, 6–7, 23, 31, 52–53
  brainwashing and, 53–54, 66–69
  courage and, 40
  macho approach to, 191–192, 205
  rape culture and, 140
Maslow, Abraham, 32
Mass media
  abstinence and, 61–62
  censorship and, 179
  challenging assumptions of, 203–204
  children and, 214–215
  complaining to, 205–211, 222–223
  and desensitization to violence, 182
  erotic versus violent sex and, 183–185
  giving positive feedback to, 208
  humor-aggression connection and, 137,
    180–181
  nonsexual violence and, 186–187
  portrayal of male behavior, 4–5

pressuring others to challenge, 209–211
rape culture and, 135–137, 178
sexual pressure and, 53–54
sexual violence in, 4, 18, 136–137,
  178–185, 186–190, 221–223
See also Books; Movies; Television
Masters, William H., 6–7, 129
Masturbation, 61, 160, 168
Mead, Margaret, 178
Media. *See* Mass media; *specific types*
Meir, Golda, 147
Men
  boasting by, 24, 67–68
  cultural messages to, 30–31, 135–137,
    178
  as involved fathers, 215–216
  macho personality in, 191–192, 205
  "nice guys," attitudes toward, 6
  as objects of sexual staring, 164
  rape of, 24, 134–135, 137, 145–148, 161
  resisting destructive images of, 206
  risks of sexual exploitation to, 5–6
  sexual coercion of, 161–162
  sexual harassment of, 5, 113, 122, 161
  sexual pressure, resistance to, 5, 6–7, 13,
    23, 38–40, 52–53, 66–69
  women's attitudes toward, 5–6
  See also Masculinity
Mental health professionals, sexual harassment by, 129
*Men Who Hate Women and the Women
  Who Love Them* (Forward and Torres),
  142
Miedzian, Miriam, 191–192, 215
Mixed messages, 21, 32–33, 58–59, 68–69
  rape and, 18, 140, 141, 147, 149–150
  sexual harassment and, 118
  about sexual intrusion, 166–167
Moral standards, 20, 177–178
Movies
  challenging assumptions of, 203–204
  debriefings for, 212, 215
  prebriefings for, 211–212, 216
  ratings for, 209–211
  realistic violence in, 193–194, 207
  sexual violence in, 4, 18, 135–137,
    186–187, 188, 209–212

Music videos, sexual content of, 4
National Coalition on Television Violence
(NCTV), 187–188, 194, 207–208,
210–211, 222
National Council on Alcohol and Drug
Abuse, 25
National Crime Victimization Survey, 133
National Institute of Mental Health, 188
National Survey of Adolescent Males, 31
New Woman magazine, 6
New York magazine, 4
Nonassertiveness, defined, 10–11
Norman, Hilary, 136
Nurses, sexual harassment by, 129–130
Nymphomania, 185

Obscene phone calls, 8, 12, 160, 168–170
hostility of, 17
jokes about, 201
treatment for, 172
Ogling, 110, 162–165

Peeping Toms, 160, 164–165
Personal fables, 85
Personality
childhood influences on, 33–34,
42–44
depression and, 44–45
Persuasion, 159–160, 161
Physicians, sexual harassment by, 129–130
Picketing, 208–209
Planned Parenthood, 97, 223
Pleasure, family scripts and, 34
Policy statement, sexual
and condom use, 90, 91
discussing, 60–61, 73–74
importance of, 58–60
rape prevention and, 145–146
Pornography
degrading features of, 189–190
erotic versus violent, 183–185
influence on behavior, 192–193
rape culture and, 136, 188, 190
sexual staring and, 164
violent, research on impact of, 180
*Pornography: Women, Violence, and Civil
Liberties* (Sweet), 185

Posttraumatic stress disorder, and sexual
harassment, 111, 114
Power
female cultural role and, 31–32
of helping professionals, 18
rape and, 8, 147
sexual harassment and, 109, 120, 128
of speaking up, 217
Prebriefings, movie, 211–212, 216
Pregnancy
abortion and, 98–99
male risks in, 5
prevention of, 97–98
sexual assertiveness and, 7–8
sexually transmitted diseases and, 63–64,
81, 82
sharing expenses related to, 17
teenage, 3, 64
Promiscuity, family influence on, 43
Protest, 193, 208–209
Psychoanalysis, 61
Psychotherapy, 229
Puberty, changes in, 19
Pubic lice, 85
Publishers Weekly, 208

Quest for Respect (Braswell), 153
Quina, Kathryn, 140

Ramos, Norma, 215
Rants-Rodriguez, Deanna, 67–68
Rape
acquaintance. *See* Acquaintance rape
alcohol use and, 24, 142, 143, 146, 151
child sexual abuse and, 152
as crime of anger and power, 8
culture of, 134–141, 164, 179
defined, 133–134
drug use and, 24
emotional aftermath of, 152–153,
154–155
extent and frequency of, 3, 133,
137–138, 190
gang, 138, 178
help immediately after, 153–154, 228
legal issues concerning, 134, 145, 151,
154, 161

male, 24, 134–135, 137, 145–148, 161
male justification of, 149–150
marital, 134, 178
mixed messages and, 18, 140, 141, 147,
    149–150
pornography and, 136, 188, 190
prevention of, 7, 145–148, 150–152, 153,
    226–228
in romance novels, 4
sexual assertiveness and, 8
sexual confusion and, 58–59, 66–67
support groups for, 46–47
survivors of, 134–135, 140, 141,
    152–155, 188, 226, 228
on television, 4
Rape, *continued*
    types of men and, 204–205
    victim role in, 8
Referrals for treatment, 206–207
Rejection, sexual assertiveness and, 72–73
Respect, 58, 63, 114–115
Rewards, 38–40
Rights, sexual, list of, 15–19, 35–36
Rowe, Mary, 125–126
Russell, Diana, 188
Rutter, Peter, 128

St. Lawrence, Janet, 57–58, 99–100
Sanday, Peggy, 134
School
    sexual harassment and, 119–122
    sexual rights and, 18
Scripts, family, 33–34, 42–44, 47
Seduction
    dishonesty and, 17, 56–57, 66, 93
    friendly professionalism versus, 116–120
    lines, recognizing, 54–57
    lines, responding to, 56, 67–72
    parental, 42–43
    See also Sexual pressure
Self-esteem, 38
    courage and, 40, 92, 144, 217
    defined, 38
    and discussion of condom use, 95–96
    masculinity and, 68
    rewards and, 38–40
    and sexual harassment, 114–115
Self-hypnosis, 45–46

Self-talk, 34–36
    affirmations in, 36, 45–46
    and self-hypnosis, 45–46
    in thought-stopping, 41–42
Sex crimes, impact on men, 5–6
Sex education programs, 19, 62–64, 216
Sex in the Forbidden Zone (Rutter), 128
Sexual abuse
    of children, 3, 152, 161
    male, 161
    risk of being raped and, 152
Sexual addiction, 17
    childhood influences on, 43
    support groups for, 46–47
    treatment for, 154, 169, 172, 228–229
Sexual aggression
    defined, 10
    "How dare you?" response and, 24
    sexual assertiveness versus, 6–7
Sexual comments, 116–117, 120, 165–168
Sexual desire, lack of, 3
Sexual dysfunctions, 3
Sexual ethics, 15–19, 56–57, 66, 93, 152
Sexual exploitation
    risks to men, 5–6
    risks to women, 6–7
Sexual harassment, 109–132
    complaining about, 124–126
    costs of, 113–114
    by coworkers, 111, 123
    defined, 109–110
    discussion of, 124–125, 127
    by employers, 109, 110
    false claims of, 5, 8, 112–113, 127
    flattery and, 116–117, 120
    guidance for handling, 115, 126–127,
        224
    by helping professionals, 128–130
    keeping records of, 124
    legal issues, 18, 127, 224
    of men, 5, 113, 122, 161
    power and, 109, 120, 128
    prevention, 127
    by professors, 119, 120, 121–122
    recognizing, 110–113
    responding to, 8, 114–126, 130–131
    seeking emotional support, 126
    sexual assertiveness and, 8

sexual confusion and, 115, 117
sexual staring, 110, 162–165
stages of, 114
treatment for harassers, 130
and uninvited sexual comments,
116–117, 120, 165–168
Sexual intrusion
coercive, 160
degrees of, 160–161
flashing, 170
noncoercive, 160
obscene phone calls. *See* Obscene phone
calls
ogling, 10, 162–165
reporting, 172–173
stalking, 171–172
treatment for sex addicts, 169, 172
uninvited sexual comments, 116–117,
120, 165–168
voyeurism, 160, 164–165, 170–171,
172
Sexually transmitted diseases (STDs)
abstinence and, 63–64
attraction and, 83, 99–100
basic principles of, 85–86
and beliefs about health, 37
cheating and, 66
discussion of, 17, 87–98
exposing another person to, 102–103
extent of, 79–83
holistic approach to, 46–47
information on, 223–224
legal issues concerning, 102–103
major, 79–82, 86–87
men and, 5
rewards and, 38–40
risks of acquiring, 3, 5, 79–87
risk triggers and, 83–85
self-hypnosis and, 45–46
sexual assertiveness and, 7, 16
testing for, 100–101
Sexual pressure, 51–75
abstinence and, 60–65
arousal and, 15–16, 65–66
brainwashing in, 53–54
cheating and, 66
customs of, 51–53
ideal sexual assertiveness and, 57–58

lines, recognizing, 54–57
lines, responding to, 56, 67, 68, 69–72
men and, 5, 6–7, 13, 23, 38–40, 52–53,
66–69
policy statement and, 58–60
rationality and, 53–54
rejection and, 72–73
resisting, 15–16
women and, 6–7, 52–53, 69–71
See also Seduction
Sexual rights, list of, 15–19, 35–36
Sexual staring, 162–165
Simon & Schuster, 208
Songs, 4, 18, 53
Spiegel, David, 45
Spiegel, Herbert, 45
Stalking, 171–172
Statutory rape, 18, 129
Strauss, Susan, 112
Stringer, Gayle M., 67–68
Support groups, 46–47
Surgeon General's report, 180
Survivors, 135
Sweet, Corinne, 185
Symptoms of STDs, 80–82
Syphilis, 80–82, 102

Teenage pregnancy, rates of, 3, 64
Telephone calls, obscene. *See* Obscene
phone calls
Television
children and, 214–215
music videos and, 4
sexual violence on, 4, 18
violence on, 187–188, 194, 207–208,
210–211, 222
Testing for STDs, 80–82, 102 (also see
Appendix)
Thoughts, rights to sexual, 16–17
Thought-stopping, 41–42
Tone of voice, 20–21
Transforming a Rape Culture, 204–205,
209
Trichomoniasis, 85
Trust
and helping professionals, 18
between men and women, 5–6
rape and, 135, 141

self-esteem and, 38
sexual ethics and, 17, 56–57, 66
sexually transmitted diseases and, 17

Uninvited sexual comments, 116–117, 120,
    165–168

Vander Waerdt, Lois, 126
Vintage Books, 208
Violence, sexual
    and attitudes toward masculinity, 4,
        6–7
    desensitization to, 182
    exposure to, 4
    gay bashing, 3
    moral outrage concerning, 177–178
    on music videos, 4, 18, 136–137
    negative effects of, 186–190
    pornography and, 190
    in print media, 4, 18, 136–137
Violence, sexual, *continued*
    in television and movies, 4, 18, 135–137,
        178–187, 188, 209–212
    See also Acquaintance rape; Rape

Virginity, 23–24, 30, 52, 61–62, 65
Visualization, 41
Voyeurism, 160, 164–165, 170–171, 172

Warshaw, Robin, 141–143, 144
Webb, Susan, 111
Wolter, Dwight Lee, 64
Women
    clothing rights of, 18–19, 118, 141, 149,
        163–164
    cultural messages to, 31–32
    and macho personality in men, 192
    powerlessness and, 6–7
    risks of sexual exploitation to, 6–7
    as sexual objects, 4, 7, 17, 150–151,
        162–165, 165–168
    as victims of sexual pressure, 6–7,
        52–53, 69–71
Women Against Pornography, 184, 215

You-statements, 22–23

Zillmann, Dolf, 189